Health,
a Conscious Truth

A true labor of love.

Diana Andrew

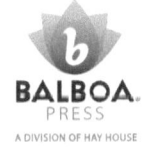

BALBOA.
PRESS

A DIVISION OF HAY HOUSE

Balboa Press books may be ordered through booksellers or by contacting:

Balboa Press
A Division of Hay House
1663 Liberty Drive
Bloomington, IN 47403
www.balboapress.com
1-(877) 407-4847

Because of the dynamic nature of the Internet, any web addresses or links contained in this book may have changed since publication and may no longer be valid. The views expressed in this work are solely those of the author and do not necessarily reflect the views of the publisher, and the publisher hereby disclaims any responsibility for them.

The author of this book does not dispense medical advice or prescribe the use of any technique as a form of treatment for physical, emotional, or medical problems without the advice of a physician, either directly or indirectly. The intent of the author is only to offer information of a general nature to help you in your quest for emotional and spiritual well-being. In the event you use any of the information in this book for yourself, which is your constitutional right, the author and the publisher assume no responsibility for your actions.

Any people depicted in stock imagery provided by Thinkstock are models, and such images are being used for illustrative purposes only.
Certain stock imagery © Thinkstock.

ISBN: 978-1-4525-5421-1 (sc)
ISBN: 978-1-4525-5422-8 (e)

Library of Congress Control Number: 2012910964

Printed in the United States of America
Balboa Press rev. date: 09/11/2012

Contents

Dedication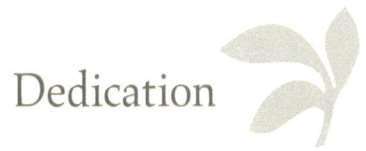

I dedicate this book to all struggling in their journey to good health. May you find a sense of being understood and heard through the writing of this book.

I also want to dedicate this book to my mom, for if it was not for her understanding of how important it was for her children to have a childhood in the mist of tragedy, this book would not have been written. Thank you for remembering the importance of our laughter and play, for our silliness of our childhood that still needed to take place. Thank you mom for staying through with your commitment to raising all of us eight children after daddy died. Thank you for knowing that our childhood was still of good use and there was Life left after his death. Your strength and dedication to raising us will not be forgotten.

May all who have lost find Life again.

LIFE IS.....

"Life is short or so I have been told and I believe it more and more every year. In that life one has to be educated, find a wife, raise a family, educate that family, get a job, and struggle. Nothing ever existed during a life even though it is short that did not have struggle. The enjoyment in life is the struggle. No struggle no life, the greater the struggle the richer the life.

There will come a time dear children when you will meet yourself getting up in the morning. You will get up, eat breakfast, go to work, eat lunch, come home, eat dinner, and go to bed. You will be surrounded by people at work and you will be surrounded by people at home. You would like to go off into a corner by yourself just to be alone. You will know that you are not getting anyplace and you will feel that you never will. You will swear that you couldn't think creatively if you had to.

You will try to think of bright ideas. What you wouldn't give for one idea that would make you rich and famous. You will feel that you are on a never ending treadmill and worst of all you will not be sure what you are waiting for.

You will look at government and war and people. You will watch people bicker over their own interests and you will hear all of the pessimists and do gooders of the world proclaim that they and only they know what the world needs.

Now dear children, may I make a suggestion to you. I would suggest that you look out and see a hill, a tree, a field. If you cannot see them then just remember they are there. There is nature. There is dirt. It has been here for a long time. It is orderly. It follows definite laws. It can be trusted. From this you will know there is order in this world in which you live. Looking out at those clouds in the sky you will know that there is purpose. You will realize that it may be beyond your understanding but this must not matter.

It is strange how this will sneak up on you. Don't ignore it children, and don't miss it. Some people jump off bridges because they miss it.

I so hope you will understand. There is always hope and always strength and always belief. I suppose that is the secret of life itself. Hope, strength, and belief.

Earl Andrew 1934-1974
Thank you Daddy.

Health, Revolutionized

This book will revolutionize the way people think about health. It will fill the gap where the intellect cannot go. It will tap into the hearts and minds of people like no book has before.

We have yet to revolutionize our hearts and minds in our approach to health, but that time has come. To heal first will be the mission of health. The miracle of healing in this book will have a profound effect on many levels for people of any age. This is a book about fundamental health, revealing deep truths about self-development, inviting people to stand face-to-face with their health in a way they've never seen or considered before. This new way of addressing our health could prove to be one of the greatest advances in real freedom.

Foreword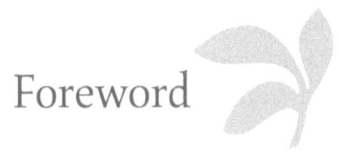

I was seven years old when my father died. I quickly adapted to the loss; that's what children do. However, as I got older, the effects of that loss began to surface. It seemed that the memory of my father became the motivating factor behind much of what I did. A deep part of me still wanted to please him and make him proud, even though he was no longer physically here.

Except for his loss, my childhood was normal. I had friends and was close with my family, and I participated in sports and activities in school. Yet I quietly suffered from this void inside. The loss of my father created an emptiness that as I got older seemed to get harder to deal with. It was my belief that since time had past and more time had past that it should somehow have taken away this void. I tried working hard at any job I did—hoping that somehow, the void would be filled by good behavior or a diligent, soldier-like attitude. I believed that if I followed well enough all that I was told to be successful as a person that it should solve this emptiness and that because of my effort everything would be fine someday.

When loss occurs at a young age, a child grows up differently. For me, it was a subtle difference, and mostly an internal one. I spent most of my life between the ages of seven to thirty still attached to my father—and that felt normal to me. Whatever I was doing, I carried both the memory of my father and the pain of his loss in the background. I didn't really have *me* in my own life. I experienced everything simultaneously through two distinct visions: one of loss, which I tried to honor each day and one of life, which I respected. The motivation behind the reason why I did anything was held in the light of my dad..

My father was forty years old when he died of a sudden heart attack, leaving a wife, four sons, and four daughters behind. Amazingly, he had written a philosophical memoir before he died; my mom gave each of the eight of us a copy when my youngest sibling turned seventeen. I would read it quite often, crying much of the time. My father was wise and would have offered great counsel for his children had he lived, so I sought guidance through his written words.

One afternoon, as I started to read the memoir, I felt water dripping down from my ear. I knew I wasn't crying; the tears seemed to be coming from somewhere else. I wiped the tears away from my ear and neck and put the memoir down. Then I went into my bedroom, shut the door, and closed my eyes.

I began to breathe deeply. After a few long deep breathes, I began to feel a powerful force of energy inside my body. This force presented itself to me as something to pay close attention to. Don't move I thought, I need to sit still and listen. The forceful presence communicated to me admonishing me to let go of my father in order to be truly free. I felt my father there, too, telling me he loved me, but I needed to let him go *now*. I was afraid to have to make a decision between my father and what felt seemed like God and self. I was afraid to let go of my father. I loved him—I couldn't do that! Yet even as I was aware of that, the powerful energy began to shake out of my thought and told me I was here to create change. Oh my gosh, this is real. I cannot argue with this at all. Although I did not know what that meant at the time, I knew that the voice meant business and that I must listen. I also knew that not letting go would continue the suffering that had been lingering in me all those years, so now was the time.

That night I went to sleep and had the most powerful dream, a dream that I will not ever forget. I was looking down from above, seeing myself next to a broken bike, which was leaning against a tree. This bike I recognized as a bike that had been given to our family by a unanimous person that cared about the well being of our family. The bike was somewhat rusted, the green paint had been chipped over time, but in our family that bike represented freedom. As I was seeing myself next to the bike, wondering what I was going to do with it a presence next to me asked me if I could fix the bike. I said that I could try, but really in my heart, there was know way I would be able to do it. Then the presence asked if I could fix the bike to look like —and I was shown a bike that was the same make and model but brand-new, with no marks or dents, no dirt or broken parts. This bike though was pure white. Now I knew I couldn't do that, so I said no, I didn't think so. The presence said to me if I was willing to follow, I would be shown how to fix the bike. So, from then on I have been on a ride of a life time.

Losing my father and coping with the resulting void had left me unable to find a path to good health that worked for me. For years I did not realize that my early loss had created such deep suffering in my life. Letting go of the loss, and my attachment to the relationship I had maintained with him after his passing, was the beginning of the *new* beginning of my life. That's how this book started.

After all the whirling of information, diets and exercise plans, I was very aware that we still don't know what health is. There had been something missing completely from the picture. And it is when I asked for the truth of what was missing in health and why we are still asking what to have for breakfast as grown adults that I received this huge opening. Mind you, this has not been easy, but it has been worth it and continues to be worth it.

I don't own the path to healing or health; nobody does. Healing lies between the soul and God, not just with the intellect. By claiming the rights to healing or health through information alone, we resign ourselves to continued suffering. We must trace back our own personal history over time, not just the physical history, but the mental, emotional and spiritual history as well in order for healing to take place within us and on the planet.

I feel very fortunate to have received guidance from this presence. The manuscript began from one simple question, what is health? From that question I listened for the answer. The question began to answer me whenever I would finish working out. I would take a pencil and the paper they had supplied on the counter, sit down and listen and write. Then I would go home and continue for a while. Usually it was about a 2 hour time period just about every day but weekends. My sister Kathy, would see my coming up the stairs, I would walk in and she would say," I know Diana I can't talk to you because you need to sit down at the computer and type." And my reply would be," sorry Kathy, but this is what I have to do". When I would wake up in the morning, I would check in to see would it be the mind, the body or the spirit. Which one? I never over worked the mind, the body or the spirit, there was a rhythm that started to take place. Each needed to be addressed in a positive, constructive way. The writing would go on at work too. I would be waiting tables and still be aware to keep my ears open during slower periods. Even my coworkers would say, "Oh, there she is writing again". It did not bother them, they seemed excited to know there was something brewing up stairs. Eventually after about 4 years the writing stopped. It was done, I would check to see if there was anything left and sure enough, that was it. The rest is history.

When you see the Life spelled this way, it is referring to the power beyond us all. It means there is something greater than ourselves that we may want to consider when things happen beyond our "control". Health is spelled with a capital H as a reminder that Health is a power within its own self. It is not in power drinks, anything advertised or man made, it is the function of your system, it is beyond once again anything you could imagine. It is like the Father of all Father, like the Godfather of the body. It is something that needs to be respected and honored showing our reverence for Life. The system of the body has the highest reverence for Life and persons, if we show the same respect and appreciation in return, there is a beauty in that.

What I am sharing in the pages that follow is the wisdom I received from the presence of Life and Health. Reflecting now upon the time spent receiving this knowledge, I am aware that it came from the source that is consciousness itself. It is in you it is in me and we can have a guided relationship with this consciousness, in fact that is what it is for and yet we skip over it believing our intellect is the carrier of all that, no, it is consciousness itself that is the carrier of all that is. My hope is that these words ignite some fire, some inspiration for anyone suffering, afraid to go beyond what they have always conceived themselves to be. To rise beyond and know that there is freedom and they are welcome and worthy of it while they are here. You don't have to go to the great beyond to be free, you can be free right here, right now.. May this book become a springboard to your own deep connection with Life and may it expand you awareness of what it really means to be healthy.

When Life Is Governed, Freedom Is Lost

Neither our life nor our body was designed to be governed, for in the governing of either, freedom is lost immediately. We become prisoners to the life being governed or to the body that has forgotten its freedom. Either one is tragic to the soul.

I believe it is not possible to fully realize what it means to be alive, or to discover and understand how the body functions, with all its complexities. But by getting to know ourselves better, we give our bodies a better chance of survival.

Maybe you can remember a time when you were most free, when you felt an undying freedom. This memory exists in all of us if we are willing to sit in deep reflection of our past. If you can recall such a time, if you feel that the freedom was real, you can call it back again and it can do nothing but come back. —at any age, at any time.

Children unknowingly and naturally stay open to Life for as long as they can, until they start to hear and listen to the governing of "life." The pressure to succumb to those around them who believe they know better becomes so powerful that children slowly let go of their freedom, letting go of who they are.. They give in to the movements and distractions surrounding them, believing that what they are witnessing is Life. Fortunately, the freedom you had as a child to dream and to live Life is still here. It can never leave, because the Life that courts the young child never leaves; it simply gets covered over. That very life that wants to return to you once again stays close, knocking every now and then hoping you will open the door to it.

For most of us, life has become a matter of doing, and the doing is connected to more doing, but yet there may not be real reason as to what and why, yet we are burning away life, our energy for what? Through all our doing, Life cannot connect to us; we are always running from it, tuning it out as we do this and that, thinking everything we need and want is "out there" instead of *in here*. Poor health happens when we run away from Life instead of toward it. There is a guide within all of us; however, that guide is not man. Our biggest blunder in life is following each other and not the strongest, most powerful guide—the one within us. If someone can't even see who he is inside, how can he show someone else the way? How foolish we have become.

If you are looking for health, at some point you will have to let go of the governing that has become your life and your body. You'll have to trust in what has not yet been shown in order to have your health and your life back. If you are following anyone or anything, you are not following your life!

Life connects itself intimately with children, knowing eventually they will be pulled away by others as their wide eyes look trustingly up at those around them for guidance and support. Therefore the time that Life has with every child is very precious. It is a brief period when Life can lay its gentleness upon them while they are playing in the cool of the afternoon. Have you noticed how children often get quiet when they play? As they play, there is something settling and calming them; the soft, delicate beauty from the outside matches the original grace and sweetness within them, and there is peace. For the briefest moment, it is a genuine reflection of Life upon life.

In children you see grace, beauty, love, and wonder. That is Life. Yet children lose that Life along the way. The outside governance of their minds and bodies takes hold, and they begin to live less and less authentically, less in keeping with their true nature.

Watch a child discovering new things: that is Life courting life. Watch a child at play, and you will remember Life doing the same to you. When we get older, children can help us recall what Life feels like. And learning to respect the time that Life has with children—allowing that relationship to take place unencumbered—would be a great justice to them, the best gift to give our children. Soon they, too, will get swept away by the world of doing; they will forget until they try and remember the time when life felt good to them. Life won't have changed its relationship with them, however; they will have changed their relationship with it.

Now let us move from Life and children to the body and children. Most kids love to play and dance— they simply have fun in their bodies. They will jump around and spin for what seems to be no reason at all. But this play has a purpose; it helps children get familiar with their bodies. (How does it feel to stand on your head? To move your leg this way or that?) They are free, they feel it and know it! By playing, children are learning in the moment and developing a relationship with their bodies. This is healthy and good for them, and it is their right. Maybe one of the first rights children have is to play ungoverned by any human being in the world.

Important things often go unnoticed, and play is no exception. It lays an important foundation in children's physical, mental, emotional development. That is why kids behave as they do when they are young; play is innate in them. It is a time when they are laughing, their whole soul is engaged in whatever it is they are doing. The body knows this, and maybe the child does, too—play feels good to them for a reason. Looking back to my own early childhood, I sensed that my life would soon get more serious, so I should enjoy it while I could. As a child I loved taking in deep breaths of air, smelling the summer heat as it baked on the pourch. The crisp winter air, that made my nose run and my face feel frozen. The spring air meant school was almost over, hate to say it but I loved the smell of spring. Fall always reminded me of Christmas being just around the corner, as a child who does not love Christmas?

The body was not designed to compete with our intellect, it is way more advanced. Rather, the body was made to be in uniform to the rhythm and flow of Life. Now with technology being used so much, the bodys' rhythm is really being thrown for a loop. There is no rhythm. Unfortunately, we have created an unseen battle between the mind and the body that actually undermines health's natural power. The fall away from health and our natural connectedness with the body begins when we are children, when we aren't allowed to be just who we are—curious, open, questioning everything. Our movements are free when we are children and as time goes by, the free movement becomes more about movement of right or wrong, good or bad. Questioning ourselves now and trying to align ourselves with everything we have been told is so exhausting and a drain. As we become adults, we are educated with false "truths" about life and health. And somewhere along the way, a break occurs in the connection between the mind, the body, and the spirit. I believe that the break is due in part because we have stopped trusting ourselves, doubt starts to settle within about who we are. All three were connected beautifully when we were born, but they split apart because Life was not enough in and of itself, each child seems not to be enough in and of themselves. With that comes the constant need for something other than what you already have inside. In essence, our intellect has managed to disconnect us from ourselves, to disconnect our body from Life. In effect, we are trying to piece together what constitutes healthy living with fragments—information from a conglomerate of outside sources—while true health is simply a matter of being once again.

There isn't one person who has not experienced this separation. In fact, most people go to their death still separated from themselves and the Life that was designated for them to live. It is not easy to pry ourselves from the path society carves out for us. However, the path we should follow is found within ourselves, not in the society. The society is constantly changing itself. It is designed as a symbol of all of us changing and growing and evolving, however it does not represent who each individual is, only the individual can do that..

As we grow up, we slowly abandon ourselves and the connection we have to Life in order to move outward, toward what we are told is our rightful place in this society. We unconsciously choose to invest in the societal view rather than what Life would have for us. Is this true for you? Do you want to take a new path, one that will help you find yourself again? Would you like to be in a place in which the world is moving, but you are no longer wound up in it as if your life depended on it? In this other place, it is truly possible for you to begin your life again.

At some point, we have to trust ourselves to live the life we feel called to live, even when we feel pressured by a society that may think differently than we do. . I always say that if you are not on a path, you are all over the place—and if you've chosen to follow the society, consider yourself all over the place. If you don't choose your life, then your life will be chosen for you. You will get what the society is harping on in the moment, you will get what society deems important, which is just the ones that choose to speak out, it may not be the majority, but they are the ones speaking so they are the ones heard. Choosing your life, and not just going along with the one the people of the society deem is the cause , is not easy. You have to remember, before the society ever changed, and as the society keeps changing your calling, your reason for being here was already decided and it had nothing to do with the society.However I feel each calling or reason for each person being here is in line with what the society may need at the time for the upliftment of humanity, so that those coming into the world have a better chance of continuing on with what is already decided upon by Life itself. We are just helpers here raising the concsciousness one generation at a time. Getting back in line with your destiny and stepping away from the pull of all that you have been told will require that you think for yourself and fight for the life you envision, trusting the guide within you to show you the way. The beautiful thing about the guide within us is that it benefits all of life, not just the individual. So following it is in no way selfish. Even though it is found within you and guides you, it is helpful to those around you, too. Eventually, with that guidance, your Life becomes what you are actually living, and it takes flight. Then the fighting ends: you are one with the guide once again, and the guide is one with Life.

When we're separated from the life we meant to live, we stop trusting ourselves. We begin to give our life up to the experts' opinions of what constitutes health, because we now view health through our broken and fragmented vision. We have become a people afraid and confused which is a dangerous thing when we have to live in this world. We're conditioned to leave the knowing to the experts, and to believe in them, when in reality, the knowing is within all of us. Granted, it is much easier to agree that everything is okay if the experts say it is,rather than seeing things for ourselves, which requires us to look at life from a different angle. We are consciousness, but yet very few are conscious that is the problem. We have to wake up and not be afraid of who we are and what we can become!

Poor health is a sign that we have placed our own personal responsibility of taking care of ourselves onto whatever comes by. Now I know that sounds harsh. But let me ask you," Would you just drop your car off to any person, leaving it to them to take care of?" well that is what we have done with our own health. We are meant to live within ourselves, not outside ourselves. We are meant to take personal responsibility of ourselves. When we give up that we give up our consciousness of ourselves of our lives each and everyday!! It is the living outside ourselves that has made us afraid to live. If we're aware of this, we can begin to heal the cracks within us evenly and thoroughly, using as much time as we need. Admitting that you are broken is the most loving thing you can do for yourself and for the repair of your soul, because it puts the power back into you and draws you closer to your soul, where a healthy relationship can be possible. In health it is not what you do, but the bravery in which you have to live!!

The fall happens because we've forgotten that we are born whole, we barely had a chance to taste this is when we were young. Information does does not make you whole, you make you whole.. It takes a strong person to get healthy inside, because Health doesn't play the silly society game; it is not about a look of any kind.. Health plays Life's game, and Life takes each person as she is, not discounting anything. Life already has everything—all it needs is you. And if you have IT and it has you, then you realize that everything you want you already have. But yet you have been told over and over again that you don' t have it yet, you have to have this now or that now. Always it is something, it never ends . Real life does not exist in what you can see; it exists purely in the growth of the soul. Life uses the society as its game board, putting things in place each day to help a person grow, learn, and see. Life is conscious always it is conscious, it is always trying to make us conscious, until finally we are in conscious union with it and it with us. It is great!! Life is all for the benefit of the person and his soul. However, if we believe we don't exsit yet because we don't have a certain amount of money in the bank, or because we don't have this kind of body, we will never feel as though we exist. The human race was not born with money, they were born with a soul and that is what we have to get back to, first and formost. If we put our value in what we do which is changing every single moment of the day we will never find ourselves as whole. However if we put our value in the fact that we are human beings and that in and of itself is a gift, we will be doing ourselves a huge favor.

I am not sure if anyone has noticed, but we humans have a collective pattern of consistently discounting and discrediting ourselves. It is important to recognize this so we can stop this pattern; otherwise our lives and our efforts will have meant nothing. Everything we do means something in the eyes of Life, and Life does not discount or discredit any of us in any way.

The pattern of discrediting our lives and ourselves starts at a very young age, when we learn that the things important to us don't matter in the adult world. In essence, we're taught that our life doesn't exist yet, or it won't exist until this or that happens, so we are consistently living with things that need "doing" so we can have life. Thus begins our separation from ourselves and our Life at the youngest of ages, until the separation eventually becomes permanent—and the forgetting becomes complete.

Why does this happen to all of us? Because we are afraid to be left behind in the world. We have been taught that life happens outside of us, and we have left nothing within us; we've given away our souls to anything of promise. Yet those that win the world lose their life in it, and those that keep their life lose the world. It is a choice we all must make. One credits the world and discredits Life, while the other discredits the world while crediting and acknowledging Life. We must find the balance between the two in order for Health to thrive within us.

As the child becomes distant from his own consciousness, the child soon learns not to live from the fundamental energy of his being (his soul), but from the energy of his thoughts. He slowly adapts to being governed by his own mind. Which has been replaced by the governing energies of his thoughts. Soon, he is living without the energy of his soul, which has been replaced by the energy of his thoughts. However, his thoughts are not who he is; they were never meant to have power over Self.

Ultimately we forget that freedom ever existed. Life already knows our true nature, and so does the body. If you can recall the strong connection to the freedom you once shared with Life and your body, you will be able to restore all that was lost. The bond that Life creates with a child never breaks. Childhood is the most special time of our lives, the purest, the most fun, and the simplest of times. As adults, we can live in that place without compromising worldly success in whatever we choose to do. The beautiful thing about this way of living is that we are not sacrificing ourselves anymore; we are living without governance of the self by thought or mind.

Eventually children come to believe that freedom comes from getting things, having things, and doing things. The freedom they once had slowly slips away as they become more like us and watch us become less of ourselves. This outward turn leads to the death of every child's soul and the extinction of the Life destined to live.

Are we witnessing the extinction of Life, having routinely given our souls away so freely, as if they had no value to us at all? A person who gives away his soul also relinquishes his mind, body, and spirit, for the soul is connected completely to every aspect of the person; the soul is in the mind, the body, and the spirit. There is no place the soul is not! You must not give your soul to anyone or anything, for that's what guides you through this life—give that away, and you sink.

We must believe we are sufficient for life just as we are. Therefore, it is time we take back our souls. For too long, we and our children have watched with confusion as the life we thought we knew melted down into mere physical matter. Is that what we want to believe about our lives? Is it what we want our children to believe about theirs? Our children must understand that their heritage is not what we tell them it is; it is what they believe it is, inside themselves.

I do not want to see the extinction of Life on this planet, but in not doing anything to reverse that process, we are damaging lives that are meant to be lived. I believe we can unlearn this backward way of living and finally move toward what we have not yet learned in order to live Life again.

We have been guided, as are all children today, not to the freedom that already exists within us, but to what we call "freedom" based on our ignorance of Life. Out of that ignorance, we race through life fearfully, having abandoned our soul to the ways of man instead of living through our faith in Life. Fear wreaks havoc on the soul, while faith creates peace there.

Life knows we are trying to govern it because we have learned not to trust it, to be afraid of it. The more we try to control Life, the more we fear losing it. That is why Life connects with the child as much as possible: the young child is practically without fear. We should treasure and protect this time of childhood, and we should not interfere with it, for Life is nurturing the child, spoiling her with its energy.

Life never forgets the time spent with anyone while he is open and free to enjoy it, as nothing can erase Life's memory of any one of us, no matter our age. One childhood memory—one memory not governed by the outside world, given to you by Life itself—is enough to call freedom back into your life. The impression this moment leaves within each child is sacred to him, evoking a time of connectedness with Life, a time when he was special to Life and Life was special to him, a time when he had dreams and the freedom to live.

Now is the time to regain Life, to regain your freedom. In doing so, your life will be as healthy as it was in the beginning. You can slowly recover within you the freedom that was taken away as your soul became governed. Real freedom, the freedom you felt when your Life was courting you, can never go away.

Try reflecting on this period of your life. You *can* gain back what appears to be lost or missing. Tap into that memory as much as you can, and soon you will have Life again as you used to experience it. Physically and emotionally, you will be back in that place where life was beautiful, where peace and happiness were abundant, where you knew how Life was supposed to feel.

Chapter 1

The Body as Consciousness

Exercise is important for the maintenance of the body. Unfortunately, we have reduced exercise to a means to achieve a certain "look"—so much so that we overlook the simpler purpose exercise should be used for.

What we need in this country is to empower ourselves with the attitude of *Yes*, I know what to do to lose weight. *Yes*, I know how to exercise. *Yes*, I can do it. Instead of relinquishing our power to effect personal change, giving our power away to things, people, or places outside ourselves, we can learn to do it ourselves. There is a time and the time is now that we need to be conscious of ourselves, not self-conscious but conscious that we are here for a purpose and that life is real, beyond the body.

The first step in empowering yourself is taking time for reflection and contemplation, asking yourself questions only you can answer: *How did I come to feel so bad about myself? How did I manage to gain so much weight?* How did the disconnect between me and my body happen? At this point in the process there is no need to get on the scale, no need to find a new diet. Diets and exercise plans do not address these very important and empowering questions. So before you sign up for a gym membership or try to change anything about yourself, ask yourself to whom you have given away your power. Could it be your husband? Your kids? Your community? How you have been told you "need" to exist in the world, or else?

We do not know how important empowering ones own self in this country is. Each one of us is consciousness. Consciousness lives within all of us, if we do not check in with it and trust it, then we loss it. The feeling of loss of our consciousness, that wakeful part of ourselves that is always trying to catch our attention, is what is meant to live. If by not living out of our own state of consciousness, we only know that we do not deserve to feel wonderful about ourselves until someone *says* we are wonderful after we have performed for him or her, like a monkey in the circus. We have been led to believe in all sorts of people, places, and things other than ourselves.

Our life's destiny is not to know our bodies, but to know ourselves. It was not our actions that created any of us, nor was it any use of a word. The continued belief that we have to do something special to feel our existence, or that we have to always find the proper words to say in order that we can exist in the world is a complete story that has been going on for a long time. We are not obligated by any means to keep this story going. We were all created in silence, our existence came by way of the birth canal and yet we feel as though we owe everyone our life and our self. Words cannot change what has been created, so we are now being asked to live in the creation that we are. Not to recreate the creation but to live in the creation at this time.

This quest for our consciousness is not found in the physical body, even though that has been the route we thought was all that existed. The route to consciousness the route to health is found in the persons own ability to develop a relationship with themselves, not with their body. The connection through exercise is important because it keeps you connected and respected within your own relationship to yourself. That is good. That is when you will begin to see yourself as you are. Your power lies within the self, not the body. The more powerful you are the more comfortable your body is with you, because you now get what the relation is to be between yourself and your body. The body's purpose is to stay healthy so that the person inside it can have a good life. If we choose to focus solely on the body, and not on *ourselves* in the body, we will continue to be stuck—almost as if we were buried alive.

We have to learn to see health as a matter that goes beyond our body and into ourselves, realizing that we are consciousness itself. Each one of us. Our body is consciousness, yes, but now it is time for us to be consciousness. It seems our body is letting go of that job and giving it to us so that we can thrive even more in the world around us.. Poor health comes, in part, from fear—fear of each other and ourselves, as well as fear and uncertainty about life. We live in a world in which everything is part of a system; we have systems of parenting, of education, of marriage, of religion, of government, of just about everything. Nevertheless, these systems were never meant to replace self-development. Systems are limited in their ability to sustain human life; that's not their job. So we all must decide for ourselves whether we want a life sustained by a system or one sustained by our own power. Although we may not be able to persevere without these systems, we must learn to reach further than what they offer us, realizing that we can do more on our own than what we have been led to believe.

If we can learn to break out of the need for systems, and break into a life of our own making, we will see many different changes. A good life was never meant to require a lot of money. It was never meant to be hard to reach for some and not for others. That's a bunch of baloney. Life is meant to be lived and enjoyed by everyone, regardless of what she may or may not have. We were never meant to be captured by the world; we were meant to be free, to live and be as we are called and meant to be. The world's "systems" were never intended to be the only way we defined ourselves and our lives. Sure, it's easy to fall into systems and pretend that everything is okay. When you are in line with a system, it is undemanding and cozy. It does not ask much of you, and you get what you expect from it, but where is the life in that? Don't waste your life immersed in the cushy and cozy. That's not why you are here. Find out who you are and what you are about. We can no longer live less than we are.

You are not a system of anything. You don't exist according to what others say to do or not to do. Every human being needs to experience herself and her own life based on her own truths. If we do not do that, we become ill and depressed. Don't wait around for anyone in your life. Do what you need to do, without apology. If we all did that, the world would be running nicely on everyone's inner strength and power. That would be something else!

Each of us has a truth already instilled inside us for life. When we accept this very intelligent system of truth—which does not favor things like money, fame, or itself, for that matter—we will find the freedom to live. When we go against this truth, lacking the courage to walk forward, we only hurt ourselves, creating conflict within the body and the mind, as well as the spirit. Rest assured the truth will come at us again and again, as its purpose is to develop us into strong and courageous human beings. Truth will not give up; it is determined to see us through. We just have to step forward and trust that it will catch us if we fall—and it will even allow a few steps forward just because we were willing to have faith and trust in it. In other words, believe you can, and you will!

We are supposed to know ourselves, but we cannot do that without courage. There are plenty of things in the world that can block your vision and your view, but if you keep your eyes trained on what you want, soon you will have succeeded in overcoming the things that blocked your way. Once you have done this, very little will disturb you, because you will now have what you wanted and worked hard to get: the truth about who you are and why you are here.

We are placed on earth not just to do, but to become. There is more value in someone who has the courage to become who he was born to be than in someone with a lifetime of doing and achieving.

If we decide to live a life of fun and games, we may find smiles and happiness—but they won't last long. Our purpose is to learn who we are and to do what we were meant to do, and that is how we will know true happiness. It is not easy by any means, but it does make life worth living. That is where we will find life, health, and happiness.

True, it is hard to direct yourself in a purposeful way when the world may want to pull you in many directions. But don't let that bother you; that is not your worry. Your concern should be getting to know yourself and finding out what you were meant to do. The world is filled with a lot of empty holes, holes that are meant to be filled by each person doing her part. Until we unite with our true selves, it will be close to impossible to fill in those spots, which are just waiting to be filled. Once you find your spot, your life will begin to inspire you; you will no longer feel the need to go here or there, because you will know finally that you belong.

This may not sound as though it has to do with health, but in fact it has everything to do with health. Since your body does not lie, and it is the perfect intelligent system, you will have to be truthful in your life. Follow the truth and it will lead you to the space waiting to be filled by you.

We have been taught that good health is for the benefit of the body, but only a few of us are actually getting healthy, because nobody is paying attention to how this approach to health is working. We have set ourselves up for a life of "If I do not do this, I am bad" and "If I do this, I am good." That is all wrong. We were never supposed to be caught in this cycle, *ever*. We are not our bodies, and the way we have been taught to approach health is just not good enough, not lasting enough, and a plain waste of time. Really, it is! It does not matter what you have heard about your body, about food and all that stuff. We have to recognize that health begins in our minds—and our minds are exhausted. It is time to get to a deeper level, because we are ready and we are worth it.

Get to know yourself, and you will come to find out that none of what you've been told about your health has power over you. You may be gone in a couple of years, the health-care books still sitting on your shelf, and the question will remain: Did you ever get to know yourself? Outside information has power over us only when we do not know who we are. If we get in touch with ourselves, regardless of our failings, we'll begin to understand that we were never meant to follow information as if it defined us. We were never meant to find ourselves in a workout plan written down on a page. That's not good enough for the intelligence that we are born with. It doesn't resonate with the deeper truth of who we are. Yet we follow it, because it is the only thing that we know.

Well, I want to speak to your intelligence. I want to tell you that you are wiser and more knowledgeable than what you have read, and you need to own that part of yourself in order to gain more ground in life. You are consciousness itself.

We have spent many years hiding from ourselves and others. Feeling less than who we truly are and now is the time where we are being asked to come out of hiding and into our true self, our true identity. We have regarded ourselves for way to long as just physical beings on the planet. It is now we are being asked to regard ourselves as more than physical, but as conscious beings on the planet. Therefore that goes for every child, man, woman; all that exists is consciousness. That is a big pill to swallow. In my own experience, a part of me kept wanting to deny this truth, but there is no denying it. We all exist in consciousness, not in the physical body. The physical body is here so that we recognize and see each other, yes otherwise we would not see who we are. Yet we are not what we see we are, we are more than that, we are consciousness itself!

If we continue to see each other only in the physical, than we miss who we truly our. We are divine beings, not physical bodies. We are evolving and we all must get on board with this and really trust the intuition that is guiding us. Let us not waste time on this. Health is the calling of the soul of consciousness, we cannot leave this out of the equation and expect to get well.

Going back to what is not working is wasting time. Now is the time to admit to ourselves that we know more than we give ourselves credit for. Value the consciousness that you are. We must come to realize that no amount of information will give us what we ultimately need, which is a belief in self beyond any diet, beyond what has already been written and repeated. I'll tell you, the way health tips are devoured by the public, it would seem that we are a bunch of hamsters waiting for the next feeding of information. Why? Because we have fallen away from our own consciousness and we believe that words will put everything back together again. Consciousness, quietness, silence to listen will do that. The mind loves the play of words. However, consciousness has no need for words, its wakefulness is enough in and of itself. The sun, the moon, nature is consciousness, no words; it thrives within the nature of itself and so can we.

We have come to a time in our evolution where we are going to begin to see ourselves not because of what we do, but of who we are. Our identity will know longer be tied into what we do, but will be connected to our true nature with the divine. We will begin to connect to the beginning all of which we were created in consciousness of the divine, not of the world.

What we will begin to find is that what used to work for all of us does not work anymore, because we are all evolving and to allow this change to occur without the need to control or stop it is what this energy needs in order to get us right with ourselves and each other. Truth lives within us all, we have just tuned it out and forgotten. We are now stepping into the consciousness that we are. Health will begin to exist within all of us. No longer will the information be the driving force behind our ability to change, it will be our consciousness that will guide and lead us into the change. Knowledge of health will be in our own awareness not in information, which comes and goes. That is it. We cannot continue to perceive health as the object of a lifelong battle. It has caused so much distraction and discontent in people's lives. Instead, we are to believe that we can overcome any obstacles to health, not by reading but by doing, which is how you persevere. Do not let information own you. You are not that, you were not created or born from that. You will never get to your divine true self without connecting and trusting yourself, letting go of the books. FEEL who you are!! Do not let doubt own you. Do what you have to do to overcome obstacles and own your life.

In order to feel powerful, we have to use whatever power we have, even if it is just a little in the beginning. That is fine. Health comes to someone who believes he deserves it and desires a better life than the one he has. It may not always be physically noticeable; often it's deeper than that. Understanding our lives and ourselves is much more significant than what we see, so it is important for each of us to live the life that makes sense to us and allow others to do the same. In doing so we create a sense of mutual respect while perpetuating the intelligence with which we are born. Don't let your innate intelligence die on the vine. Use everything you have to overcome your obstacles to achieving better health and you will be free, propelled by a newfound strength and determination to live the rest of your life fully. Now using the word achieve is one that I hesitate on because it may cause one to feel "against" themselves. You are in the flow of your own self now, so achieving is a term used to moving forward, breaking down emotional barriers that have been in the way. So achieving refers to one having a deeper connection with themselves.

First, you must learn what health is. You must know that before you can comprehend its power, its goodness, its necessity in our lives, we must first know what it is..

Most of us do not know what health is, so we try to comprehend it intellectually. If we understood that health resides in the connection between the person and their own soul we would see that the bigger the disconnect the poorer the health. Seeing health in this matter is wonderful and beautiful. To know longer feel we are physical objects to one another's desires, but in fact we are divine beings living and thriving on this planet for the sake of wanting better for the future beings who will inhabit this earth after us, is truly the ultimate in consciousness. That is the beauty and honor that our consciousness wants to bring to each of us and this planet if we sit, listen and take in what is being offered at this time. To put it in basic terms, all of us are to live, and the body has a job to do while that person is alive. So it is impossible to respect life without respecting the health of the body. This may seem like a radical thought, but if your body is what keeps your life going and you don't respect that, what *are* you respecting? Often we seek our own satisfactions in life without regard for our body. But health resides in the relationship between you and your body; if there is no conscious relationship, it stands to reason that the health may be somewhat poor. The life, the body, and the person need equal respect.

For if you respect your body and it starts to fail in older age, you will still be able to appreciate life. If you live without respect for your body, or you have always believed that you were your body and it begins to age, because it does and will; you may feel you have lost your life and yourself. But you didn't, and you can't—physical decline is just the natural progression of the body. It is good to understand this, as the realization of this can make life better at any age.

Doctors use their intellect to fix a body that needs repair, to figure out why the body is doing what it's doing. In the United States, we are trying to fix the health crisis through a lot of intellect and very little else. For someone to create an environment of wellness within themselves, they must first establish a new relationship with themselves. Adding intellectual mumbo jumbo can create an illusion that those who know more are better able to come to a solution; however, the solution does not lie in outside information—it lies inside us. The solution to our health problems cannot be found in a book, just like love cannot be found in the Bible, or money problems cannot be solved by money... : we have more health information than ever in this country, and more illness and disease. Fifty years ago there was a lot less information, and while we had problems, but we did have not as many of them.

We have to claim ownership of our own bodies. Because we haven't done so, we look in books and turn to doctors and nutritionists for all sorts of advice. They can give you an answer for every question out there, but the fact of the matter is, until you claim full ownership of your body, you will always be seeking more answers.

We don't seek intellectual answers regarding the care of anything else we call our own; we just happen to take care of those things naturally. Consider your house, for example: no one needs to tell you how often you should clean it before it gets to the point of being messy. You have a garden, you know that if you do this and this your plants will thrive, if you do not they will not. For us it is no different. Now, whether you want to acknowledge the truth of what needs to be done to thrive, as a human being on this planet is another thing. The knowing what to do and doing it is the key in all of this. In the same way, you don't need to ask a "specialist" when you should do your laundry or which brand of detergent is best. No, you just use your common sense. And once again, as the laundry piles up, the important question becomes, Are you going to do anything about it? Everything recycles itself. Our breath is a good example of this. Our breath does not give itself and then stop because it is to tired, or upset. Our breath is our consciousness. It is without opinion, beliefs of any sort, it is supportive and unconditional. Going back to the breath is very important for a stable and well balanced life.

The same is true with taking care of you. The answer to your health problems lies in a simple question: Have you claimed sole ownership of your body yet? Knowing that it is your sole responsibility to take care of it.

The cure for obesity and illness would be found if each of us understood that our bodies do not operate according to an agenda, and that as long as we expect them to, we will continue to pursue health to no avail. We must realize that we cannot get to the level of healing ourselves if we continue to see our bodies as images, as objects. Our bodies are not here to look good—that's not their main concern, and in fact it is not a concern of the body at all. Instead, that's our own generational history (his-her- story), which we've placed on our bodies. The body does not speak to us with words. It uses pain or discomfort as a form of communication, pure consciousness. It is that which we are, pure consciousness. By acknowledging that we are pure consciousness as our body is helps us connect to that which is all knowing, giving and abundant, which is that which lives within all of us.

Since consciousness does not have a shape or size then attaching yourself to a shape or size and saying I am that is know longer true, for you are not your shape or size, you are consciousness itself. When you make yourself a shape or size, you become that which you see yourself as. It is you that is deciding to make yourself that way. Your consciousness goes to that which you believe yourself to be. Since your consciousness is pure it takes in what you give to it as truth. This is not just for you, we all effect each other in this regard. the shape, weight, or size is not the concern of the body, we have decided to create the concern and have done quite a job doing so. We have created a full agenda for our body that directly contradicts the body. Say you have new born baby and as soon as that baby begins to walk you set your full agenda on that child. Pretty soon that child does not feel, think or do anything "naturally", it is fully running itself on your agenda alone. Well, when we set our body up like that, our body know longer runs in its natural rhythm as we are know longer in touch nor do we know what natural is. When we set our own agenda for our body, we end up losing. However, if we allow our body to do what it does best, giving it what it needs to operate most efficiently, we are free to fly, to live, to thrive.

We have to get away from thinking that we have to be the boss of our bodies, which generally does fine on its own and is far wiser and more intelligent than we imagine. Humans make the mistake of believing we are greater than our bodies until of course we get sick and then we beg our body to get well. Then we realize the value of what it means to be well and feeling good. So relax and let your body take the lead. Live and flow with your body, get to know its rhythm. Throw away the idea of body image, of size and weight. Know that you are consciousness. Let your body behave naturally. Listen to it and sense what it may need more or less of. Learn what it feels like to have a relationship with your body, without an agenda. Your body is unique to you, and therefore it will have its own special relationship with you, so just pay attention to that relationship and you will move into the next stage of learning and growing. As you continue along this path, you will come to see yourself and not your body. You will be in the world and not your body.

The body is a perfect example of teamwork, strength, focus, and love. Look at how the body systems work in with each other and you will see how a great team is put together. You will also sense and come to know how you can be part of the team without giving up feeling you have to be in control. The bodies have several major "players," like the heart, the lungs, and the stomach. If the heart neglected its function for even a second, the body might die. Again, this is consciousness; this is who we are too. We are that consciousness and wakefulness that the body demonstrates every single day. We go to sleep the body still functions and stays alive even when we are not aware. We are that consciousness, we just have to tap into that and we become that whole system of alertness and attentiveness. When we get overly involved with information, it becomes more of a distraction than anything else. It is as if we clutter up the pure consciousness that we are. The body does not neglect us we must not continue to neglect it. When we neglect our bodies we neglect ourselves because we are one in the same. When we neglect of our bodies because outside influences get the best of us, we put unnecessary strain and stress on our organs; we allow the life outside us to put the delicate balance of the working organs in jeopardy. Since the body is pure consciousness, it will never nor does it know how to live in the world and adapt to it, for it was not created by the world. So it adapts constantly to itself and that which it knows it is which is life itself. The body will not allow us continued bad choices over life itself, ever!! It will always chose life, it will always take the high road over our misuse of it. For it is obligated to life first, always life, that is it!! So the question than can be posed as this. Are you going to be on the side of life or not? Your body already is. It will not give into saying that works against the purity of life itself will one day be better. No, that will happen. So in health we must understand it is life, not a system. When you see a healthy plant, it is because it has been well taken care of. If however, the plant was not watered it would die. Now, it does not matter the kindness of who you are, that does not change the truth of what that plant needs in order to thrive. Nothing can change the truth of what that plant needs in order to thrive, if it is not given what it needs it will die. That is the state of its consciousness. The state of consciousness that we come from is the same, it is no different. If we do not do the right things in order to take care of ourselves, it does not matter the money we have. It does not matter the plans we may have 5 years from now. The body is a state of pure consciousness, it does not have the mind we have. Its mind is already made and created. If we do not abide by what it needs, we suffer the consequences. Just like the plant was made to live, and without water it dies. We are made to live, but it takes awareness and effort in order to do so.

Now let me remind you: the body is not here to serve itself; it is here to serve you. So it works super hard each day to keep up with your daily grind. But it is a two-way relationship. Your body needs you as a partner—you are the deciding factor in the efficiency and maintenance of your body. So if you are constantly in "take" mode, your body will soon respond with an altered state of health and well-being. It's up to you to appreciate and work in conjunction with your body. The body is not as strong as you may think; it does have limits to the amount of abuse and neglect it tolerates.

It is my feeling, as well as my experience, that most of us don't realize how powerful our thoughts are upon our body and how our actions create the life we live. Living in our bodies on just a physical level invites attachment. Seeing ourselves as conscious beings is important otherwise we become slaves to the attachment we have created in our bodies on the physical level. Many people live their lives in a state of passivity.

Feeling what will happen, will happen— they have no connection to their own power, their own true self, their soul. They have abdicated their power as human beings, missing each opportunity brought to them for the purpose of making that connection..

You cannot develop as a human being without wanting to become better—a better thinker, a stronger, calmer, more stable person. How can you find out who you are if you don't take responsibility for your life? What a waste of life, just living it by a wing and a prayer. Praying does nothing without awareness of what happens after the praying. If I pray for strength, the prayers response might first be that I notice my weaknesses. Oh, but when we pray we want the good and comfortable that is it. If we do not get that, then we assume our prayers are not working for others or us for that matter. In order to learn we need sometimes to look at the 'stuff' that we do not want to see. We are consciousness, when we pray consciousness hears and delivers. The taste of this medicine is powerful and often times does not taste good, our spiritual pallet is not used to what is being delivered. That does not change the delivery, it does not change what we are suppose to look at. But that does not change the fact that sometimes we have to get through the bitter to get to the sweet. for us; it is our actions that produce change. We must meet prayer with action, we must meet weakness with strength, and we must look within as we also look without. It is an equal balance of give and take. We have been given much strength; we just have not tapped into it yet. Thought without action is just thought. Actions are the wheels to change.

Know longer can the world be sustained on image alone. We have grown weak trying to gain strength from these images we have been viewing. For it is not the outside that makes a man, but the effort that he draws from the inside. Our bodies have strength and creative capability, but we must put those things into context to understand what are bodies are for, and what we are for.

So if we are going to take our health seriously, we must take it all the way, beginning with a deep understanding of ourselves. If you do not take the time for self-reflection, it will be hard to make those broader life connections.

As long as we continue to believe that only our body needs changing, we cannot get to the self inside the body that is just fine the way it is.. It is not the body that needs to change; it is the perspective that needs to change., A person suffering from illness or depression may very well be showing itself as the direct result of the distance between that person and their true, divine self. Does that make sense to you? If we are in connection with our true self that quite possible illness and disease has less of a chance to manifest within our body. Disease, dis-ease, the question may be where in your body does this dis- ease show up? Ease, dis- ease..mmm… It is very important to pay attention. Again, we are consciousness and the body does not lie, so if we chose to stay unconscious to our life and what is around us, our body still takes the truth of all that is, it is up to us to align ourselves with the truth that is presenting itself to us, always. We are in a time where each one of us is being asked and guided to take responsibility for ourselves, not because of a want or a need, be because we should.

A body cannot thrive if the person inside has made it weak. The physical body feeds off the environment of the mind and emotions, an environment that the person inside creates. Imagine a house whose inhabitant is miserable and unhappy: the house will take on the atmosphere created by the person living there. The house alone decides nothing for itself. This is critical for us to understand. While we cannot change the owner of the body, we can change the relationship between owner and the body. Seeing it now as cohabiting in such close courters that each and everything effects the balance of the other. Often times we are at the body, the body is not at us unless we cause it to be at which time it causes us to pay attention.. The bodies inherent nature is not to provide us with self-esteem, but when we choose to take care of the body in a loving way, we gain self-esteem as a byproduct of our good choices. However, if we try and create self-esteem by using our own body as a tool to gain leverage in life, in relationships, it will hurt us in the end—physically, mentally, and emotionally. Our bodies need us to take care of them; instead, we have made health into a vanity project, which is not what it is at all. Health is not about appearance. It is not a game of Do You Like Me Now? It is not an image, we are not images. You do not use your kids to enhance your image or to feed your vanity. Why? Because it is not the purpose of any person, no matter how young or old, to be used in such a way. Yet we do that to ourselves because of the images that we see all around us. It is sad that we have made the body an object, but that doesn't change the truth that we need to meet ourselves one day, each one of us, that way the image has know power over ourselves.

Your body holds you in it. It is closest to you; it is a reflection of you. The body is a reflection of who you are at any given moment. We cannot hide from ourselves, we have to see how beautiful we are. We live inside the reflection of what we believe about ourselves. What do you want your reflection to be, with that reflection it is brought out into the world each day, into our relationship each day. I hope that we can be a reflection of the divinity within, a refection of the light of our very own soul. That is the ultimate, intimate relationship one is meant to have with their body, mind and spirit, seeing them one day in the light of their own creator. Your body, mind, and spirit holds all truth, so you can lie to yourself, but you cannot lie to that part of yourself that is true. The light knows no darkness, their for if we believe ourselves to be anything less than the light, the light will be used to shine on the darkness in order for us to let go of more. Eventually we are soul, we are light, the light in which we came from, the light which calls us forth out of the darkness. It reminds us, it calls to us," listen", it says," I am here to remind you of who you are, you are that which I Am, come share in the divinity that you are."

To nurture our bodies with proper care and respect, our truest and highest nature must come alive. Then we begin to experience a reality that does not compromise for the sake of something quicker or "better." The body has a natural ability to offer instant feedback, instant reality, in its truest form.

If we can learn how to live in our bodies, we can learn how to live in the world, for there is a direct correlation between the two; what is within us is reflected in our bodies and in our lives. Living in our bodies acquires compassion, understanding, love, acceptance, the ability to accept change, and the ability to let go. You cannot be free and hold on at the same time. You are the person inside your body; your body is not you. Moreover, if you believe that your body *is* you, your body will be your master. The physical body is unemotional, uninvolved; it is the person inside who holds the emotions and is involved. However, if you make your body yourself, you burden it with expectations it is unable to fulfill. You must fill your body—it cannot fill (or fulfill) you. If you don't seek to understand yourself within the parameters of your daily life; if you don't live in the moment , then you'll seek to blame or escape. Unfortunately, our bodies often pay a price in the cycle of our resistance to that which is. Our bodies are willing to take on the burden of our lessons and learning, but there does come a time, when if we do not learn and keep making the same mistakes, the body can no longer carry itself as the vehicle and must allow the learning to take other forms of consciousness.

When we use the body to stuff our feelings or bad memories, it creates physical, emotional and spiritual suffering. Pain cannot heal through pain, it heals through love. You may think the stories you harbor from your past can no longer affect you, but if you are still holding onto them and not living fully that is a sign they are still there lingering. Are bodies are not good at concealing things that are of no use to us. Our body is consciousness itself, it does not carry baggage very well, it lives in the present moment. There comes a time when one has to figure out a better way to honor those that have passed on or to let go of feelings from the past other than holding it within their being.. If you want to have freedom in your body, you cannot keep dragging your past along with you. Your body does not lie; it's inherently truthful. The intuition within your body will tell you what to do with the stories, with the emotions you have had that no longer serve you. You just have to ask, you just have to be willing to see your body as a vehicle of consciousness of which it is. When we decide to lie to ourselves to make things appear to be okay, our body knows better, and it always goes the route of truth. It is like it has an emotional truth candle in it. It knows if you are just being a baby about something, it knows if you are being to prideful. It knows the truth of who you are and what the real deal is. So beware if you are harboring stories and at the same time wanting change to happen with your exercise plan, a new relationship, a new diet. What is underneath will still be there when you start and when you end, so find out what that is first before anything else.

That is just the way it is with health—it wants you to be free, and that includes freeing yourself from any stories you are holding on to. Now, you may be asking some questions: *Where am I to put my stories or secrets? You mean in order to have health, I actually have to let go of this baggage that I've been holding on to?*

The answer is yes—because that baggage could very well be the main cause of your health issues. If good health were just a matter of proper food and exercise, far more of us would be doing wonderfully. But your body knows the truth: there is more to health than what our intellect tells us there is.

You may wonder what's the easiest way to let go of all that stuff you have been holding inside—the effect of which your body has taken the brunt of for years now.

First, I must tell you how relieved your body will be once you let go of what you've been holding on to. And I am not talking about horrible and bad things. And if they are so be it. The worse the story and pain the more freedom will be felt, that is a good thing. There are things we all have experienced, like believing you have to be perfect, or feeling bad because you might have hurt someone's feelings awhile back. The baggage could be major, or it could be minor—it does not matter. What matters is that you're still holding on to this stuff, day after day and it is keeping you from being yourself!!

Just as alcohol does not make pain go away or change something bad that has happened, good food and an exercise plan will not change or get rid of past events that continue to haunt you. It will make you feel better yes, we are very familiar with that. But since you know your body is consciousness and so are you, that just does not fly any more. Gotta get real to be real.

The body was not meant to be a haven for everything we want to deny in life. We have to deal with our life, we have to deal with our past. Diet and exercise will not make a darned bit of difference in the long run. We have to be willing to own and be honest about what we've done, what we wish we hadn't done, or what we wish we had done but never got around to doing. Step out of denial, look at it, own it and you will be done with it. Come on, it won't kill you. What is killing you—right now—is a past that is holding you, the body that you want and the life that you dream of hostage.

Health is dealing with life on a reality basis. It will not allow you to whitewash over anything you don't want to deal with; if you want to play that game, you will get less of what health has to give. Just be honest with yourself, your body is very forgiving and will let go as you let go. Piece by piece, past by past, let it go. Since our body is consciousness it won't let you hide in it either, that is not where we are supposed to live. We are meant to live, to fly, to be free. You are the caretaker of your body, keep it clean so you can connect with its pure consciousness. We just have to get the stuff out that has been stored in it for too long.

Each person is the answer to their health problem, which, after all, would not exist but for the choices made. Therefore we cannot keep searching outside ourselves for the answer to those problems. Look within, now is the time. If our physical condition happened as a result of the choices we made, it cannot change its condition until we change our choices. If we don't decide to make healthier decisions, our health will continue to decline.

Food is not the sole factor in our health crises. If we address ourselves then the food will take care of itself. We must address ourselves or we will continue down the same path, making progress, then falling back again. We must begin by asking what is stopping us from taking care of ourselves? —a question only each person can answer. We must admit we have not learned what it means to take care of ourselves. Only then can the care begin. Before that, we might mechanically follow a food plan and exercise routine. Don't we want to feel more out of life than to mechanically follow some plan or routine? If you are following a plan I am not saying that is not the right thing to do, but learning and connecting with yourself along the way is the key to longevity and success.

Our bodies are what give us continuous quality of life. If that quality seems less than adequate, it is because we may have compromised some sort of truth we new but were to afraid to speak about it. All this effects the health we are wanting to feel and have. In order to live life with energy and clarity, we must take care of the organs that can help us do that. If our organs are clogging because of poor choices then we walk around feeling foggy and clogged, everything is connected. Good health is found in the daily choices we make —not just temporary changes because an event is coming up and we want to look good. Although that serves a purpose and there is nothing wrong with it; it is not health. What I am saying. Just so we are clear, there is a difference. All I want to do is point out the difference. *Once we learn what it means to take care of ourselves, life will take care of us and it will be such a good and even flow, the body then will not even be involved, thoughts about how you look will be know longer because you will come to know who you are which is so much more important..* When you take care of your body, your mind becomes clear, you have confidence you did not have before, and you gain an appreciation for your life, because you now sense or have experienced something different than you did before.

What could be more important than to take care of your health, when by doing so you affect the quality of the rest of your life instantly, each moment?

We cannot disassociate ourselves from our body, thinking that our body is separate from ourselves. Your body follows you around everywhere you go, it has not been separate from you since you were born. You were born together with your body, so the connection needs to be made. What is a waste of time is to want to connect to the look of someone else, that is a waste of time and energy, because that dose not work. You are suppose to connect with yourself when you are getting healthy not the look of someone elses body. Mind you people are admired for how they look, there is no denying or escaping that, but you owe it to yourself to make that connection with who you are, then you can really appreciate all the different faces and bodies, personalities and talents that embody this planet. We wake up tired and sluggish and don't bother to find out why, until eventually we have ignored our poor health for so long that we do not even notice it. Even with prescription drug use on the rise and so many people going in for surgery, people are not learning anything about themselves; they are not even wondering why they are in such poor health. And the answer to that question won't come from a doctor; it comes from within.

It is important to take the time to investigate why you are in the condition you're in. Yes, we have doctors—we need doctors—but ultimately we are the sole owners of our bodies, and we are the ones who must be held accountable for our health and learn how to live in our body.. If we lean too heavily on our doctors we will not find the real answers to our problems. For instance, if you suffer from depression, the doctor's job is not to have a long conversation about why you're depressed. So just because you leave his office with a prescription, does not mean you have found the cause of your depression. Investigate the cause before you go to the doctor; you will be doing yourself a big favor. We all must deal with issues like these from time to time—it's okay, it's not the end of the world. But let's deal with our health in the most effective way possible. Eating unprocessed foods is a start; exercising is another key factor. As you make these healthy choices, other choices needed to be made will become clear to you … and that is the beauty of taking care of yourself. When before, everything you had been doing just served to hide your feelings, now those feelings are revealed, and answers to problems become clear. We cannot reach clarity with a foggy mind and a clogged body. Working through the mud and sludge toward clear water takes time. Nevertheless, it is the most important thing that you can do for yourself.

We need our bodies, period. So it is important to take care of *you*—all day long. That simply means being aware of what you are putting into your body, putting into your mind, into your awareness. . That is it. There is no need to be consumed with anything. Just take care of your body so that it can take care of you with its vibrant beautiful life energy. You see the life in plants that are vibrant, that same life and beauty is in all of us. It is there. Good health is about being and feeling alive. If we pack our bodies with food that is "dead," we'll feel practically "dead." Low energy foods, produce low energy levels in the body, which effects how we feel, how we think. If we pack our bodies with "life," foods we'll feel alive. That is the key. Just try it out—it is not a diet. Health is consciousness of life, the one within and the one living outside of us as well.

Think about how we take care of our newborn babies: we're so careful about what we feed them and how we hold them. We are conscious of everything being brought into their lives. . But somehow once these bodies are full grown, we stop tending to them. We need to tend to our bodies with the same care and attention as we would our babies, for the same reasons. Our internal organs still need the proper nutrients to ensure good function; our brains still need to be fed so they'll work well for us. So we should maintain the simple philosophy that our bodies are just as precious and beautiful as they once were, and getting older does not mean that we can stop taking care of them. Our bodies still have critical work to do, keeping us alive. What could be more important than that? As our bodies' keepers, we have a key role in this mission, and that is how it is always going to be.

Chapter 2

Small Bite on Food

The role that food plays in our health has been taken out of context in the media. While it is true that good nutrition helps maintain proper body function, we often have unrealistic expectations of what food can do for us. For instance, ads routinely imply that eating certain foods will give you a feeling of joy and happiness. Now, no food is capable of doing any such thing. But that's what we might expect from it, because that's what we see on television. If we are empowered, we understand that such commercials are misleading, and that the products being advertised are incapable of providing all the benefits the ads say they can.

As consumers, we have gotten into the unconscious habit of believing everything we see in the media. For the sake of our health, we should empower ourselves to recognize that the relationship between the consumer and the product is one of desire and suggestion more than anything.

Chapter 3

Empowerment

The real health crisis in this country begins on an emotional level—but that concept does not sell well to the American public. Well, I suppose it does sell prescriptions. But really, we need to look at ourselves from the inside, not the outside, in order to become well.

Don't keep piling up "new" remedies for problems that will not go away. It is not the people outside of you that can fix you; it is the person inside of you that can fix you. Diet and exercise have their place, but they are a sidebar to the main story; they are not the fundamental answer to your health problems.

Gathering the courage to look within and not fear what you find there is the first step. Look, you did not intentionally place that old, worn-out baggage inside you, but now it's time to get rid of it. Let it go, and let your real life begin. Consciousness does not allow us to easily let go of the baggage, unfortunately we have to go through it and look at it, learn from it and grow. As I said, diet and exercise have their place, but your power lies inside.

As you do your internal "housekeeping," retain only what is beneficial to Life.. You do not have to give your goodness away, for example; keep it, use it, replenish it, and keep it alive inside you. Then you will experience a life of goodness, not because you eat well or exercise, but because you are you. You are you, and that is where your power is. Live off that power; it is your energy source. Nothing owns it, nothing has control over it, because it has not been created from anything outside of you.

That said, keep things in perspective. Don't do anything just to feel better about yourself, just to prove you are a powerful human being. For me, simply knowing that I was created from heaven above is enough to remind me that nothing outside needs to have power over me. Whatever the question or decision, I look inside myself for the answer that best suits me. And that is how I live.

We all need to feel successful, as if we earned or gained something that belongs to us. Without some sense of personal success in life, all we have are things and yes, of course, relationships. Most of us have attached personal success to money and things and outcomes, and we have forgotten about the reward no one can take away: the success we find on our way to a healthy body, mind, and spirit. Some people are actually turned off by the idea of success; perhaps they have no desire for money and they equate success with material gain, so that kind of success does not resonate with them. Listen, the most important success we can ever have, one that is lasting and not at all abrasive, is the success we find through self-development. That is the key to a real, meaningful life. Everything else comes and goes, and it has a tendency to breed a "give me more" mentality. However, inner success works on the development of you, and enhances your connection to life in general.

This type of personal success is vital to a happy, healthy existence. It is the success that you build on your own, from the inside, with hard work and dedication, and within the constructs of your own life. Yes, we all have to deal with certain realities and limitations. But if we bind ourselves too tightly to the ideals of success that we have been taught, where is our individuality? Where is our own personal chance in the world? Where can we find our own achievement? In our rush for worldly success, we have forgotten about our own inner success, found through the will to take care of ourselves and beyond the desire for status or material things.

Health will draw itself from the well of our inner success—although at first there may not be much in the well. In fact, it may be completely empty, having never had a drop of nourishment from you. Therefore it is your job to fill up the well by doing what you say you want to do for yourself. Each day that you wake up, you can either fill the well a little bit more, or you can choose not to. When the well starts to fill up, you'll begin drinking from the water which is now your own source of nourishment and strength. If the well runs dry, there won't be anything there when you go to it for nourishment and motivation. This filling up of the well takes commitment. Remember that what is in the well stays there, and it is always available for your personal use. In the beginning, filling the well may seem to take a lot of work, but just stay with it—you will build up inner resources that you can draw on the next day and the next, until pretty soon you'll have your own energy, your own willpower, your own power source, your own well.

If you can achieve success in your health, if you can fill that well within you to the fullest, you will have done what no one else could do for you. You are the key to your personal success; you have the power each day to fill that well and remember what you want in your own success story. The world won't fall apart if you're not paying attention to it—it will still be moving and do what it always does. So do not worry about anything external on your way to personal success.

Don't you want to see what you're made of? Aren't you curious to see how far you can go? Inner success, the success that builds character, strength, commitment, and self-esteem, is not affected by gas prices. This kind of success cannot be lost if the stock market crashes, nor can it be taxed or taken away by the government. It is not affected by the world. It is yours; you earned it, and you get to enjoy it. This is the personal success you can achieve by your hard work and dedication to your health.

If you can achieve personal success on the inside, you will come to realize that there are few things that are truly important in life, and that it is just those few things that keep life afloat and sailing smoothly. Much of what is difficult in life is unnecessary; we've done it to ourselves. Health is concerned with the basics of life, because without the basics, we don't have much. Imagine the things we rely on each day, the things we truly can't live without. There aren't many, but without them we would not last long. Health gets down to the truth about you in your body and you in your life. It's kind of like a person sitting in a small boat in a river—the boat has the river and the river has the boat, and there is not much else needed. However, you have a choice to add on and overdo—to make life more complicated, to go after all your "comforts"—or to stick to the basics: the boat and the water simply needing one another in order to reach the destination successfully.

It's exciting to strive for your own success, because you are your only competitor. You can become as successful as you want—or you can be the one to sabotage yourself. You are your boss, you are your coach, you are your instructor and your motivator, all in one. The best thing, however, is that the outcome is all yours. And remember that there are just a few things in life that are truly important. Health takes water and a boat. Stay in the boat and simply keep your oars moving. Some days may be more challenging than others in the water, but that's only because health is a process of building you up inside. Success doesn't always come easily; sometimes it takes pushing harder, and if you don't push when you need to, you will not make it. But keep in mind that health is all a matter of balance—your tougher days will lead to easier ones. Just keep going.

The journey to good health is difficult for most of us because of our perception of what constitutes strength and power. We have been conditioned by society and possibly by our religious traditions to constantly minimize ourselves in deference to those in authority. We have been trained to view authority not as a power we can use on the inside, but strictly as a power to be seen as greater than ourselves. What position do we hold in our own life if this is the view we hold throughout our whole lifetime?

Good health requires that that perception be changed. You can no longer minimize your own sense of power and authority. You are consciousness and consciousness is equal in its power within each person. Know one has the power of consciousness itself. Not to worry that this may be wrong in any way. Not using the power of our own consciousness and believing in the minimum of what we have been told is, has now changed. The continuation of this idea that we are less than someone else cannot remain in this new consciousness. In the continuation of that false truth , you will remain weak. Health a conscious Truth is about regaining the power within each of us that has been lost. Now is the time for this. The "look" of health and the "intellect" of health have caused us not to see ourselves. You must understand that your health begins by building the connection between you and your soul. When you make the connection on the inside, without your exterior appearance being the main catalyst for pursuing good health, it will all make sense to you. You will realize too, that was the piece that was missing the whole time.. We have to become strong people in our lives and in the world, and the only way to do that is to become strong in ourselves. Now by strong I am not talking aggressive. By strong I mean aware of who we are. Like a lion, look at a lion, there is know doubt a lion knows its potential, knows what is going on at all times., that is what I am talking about. We have to reclaim the power that we have relinquished to those in authority. Health requires you to retake control over yourself and your life, without controlling anything. Control in this sense means, being responsible for what you say and do, knowing that it will affect your life instantly as well as those around you. We are living in an instant society now, where there is no gap between what we say and its happening. We think technology has helped us, yes it has, but consciousness is going to trump us all.

Once you have connected to that inner authority called consciousness, you have all the power to change, to make a difference, to do whatever it is that you want to do. If you are to believe that things are suppose to happen by or through someone else, then you will wait and wait till forever for things to really change. So take ownership of your life now. Nobody but you has the authority to make the decisions that you will need to make for your health. It is up to you to decide whether you will continue to sit and waste time feeling miserable and disgusted with yourself. It is up to you to decide whether you will continue to blame others for how you feel. However, as soon as you take responsibility for your health, the journey will be easier. You will simply have to maximize the power inside you that has been minimized over the years.

It takes a powerful authority to reign over the choices that lead to full consciousness. Where consciousness is now you and you are it. You may say, what the heck does that mean. Well, consciousness is what makes the sun rise in the morning, the ocean be the ocean and within us there is that same thing. We have just lost touch with it. While you once lived passively, you now will need to make a stand for yourself each day. Blame anyone you want for your poor health, but ultimately, the one you need to scrutinize most is you. Whether your health is good or poor, you created it.

Getting back to the word *authority*: that word carries a lot of power, a confidence and a certainty that there is someone in charge. If we live with the mind-set that those on the outside claim all the authority in our lives, we will continue to feel powerless and hopeless—and no wonder! We have given away our authority our consciousness, in doing that we have instantly created a gap within us for all sorts of things to happen. Fear, anxiety, doubt, insecurity, which stands to reason. The remedy, however, is simple: we must reclaim our own authority our consciousness. Listen to it, follow it and trust it., Recognizing that we are the decision-makers, that we have the power in our lives. If we do not know and acknowledge that, of course we will feel defeated.

It is my hope that every person in the world will take a stand for his own health and understand that medical care is meant for emergencies, not as an alternative to taking care of yourself. That is really the only way that we can be effective in our lives and in the lives of our children: by teaching them how to balance their family, work, and health by making positive choices in their lives.

Do not let anyone else decide what is best for you and your health: decide for yourself what is best. Fit in exercise, fit in healthy eating— make them a priority in your life, because it is essential to our bodies that we eat well and exercise.

Your health is a reflection of how you take care of yourself. It does not belong to your neighbor, your friend, your husband, your wife, your mother, or your father. The person who takes care of herself takes care of her life properly in all areas. This is not to say it prevents problems from happening or situation from being difficult, however, it will help you to see what is real what is false, what is worthy and what may not be. Health cannot wait around for you to have time to attend to it; you don't see life waiting around until you are good and ready to live it, do you? Life goes by, whether or not we are ready for it. It does not wait for anyone.

When you are in good health, you enjoy enormous benefits—not because you lose weight or look better, but because there is an honest relationship going on with your life, and that's far more valuable. Many people develop health problems by neglecting the voice we all have inside, the one that guides and protects us, is our consciousness. It is not male or female, young or old, it is timeless and is with us throughout our whole life. Unfortunately we have fallen into the unconscious notion that if we done what we have been told than all will be well, It does not work that way, we are human and life is alive and always changing, that is what we need to be aware of. If you speak and live in your truest, highest state of mind, honoring and obeying it, you will become healthy. When you listen to that voice and take care of yourself, you start receiving more in life. You'll receive the things you've been praying and asking for, the things your life has had a hard time giving you because you kept choosing something else. A critical part of receiving the help you have asked for is to listen to your conscience, which never misguides you and never wants less for you than you truly want for yourself.

Consciousness is connected to life—every hour and every moment—consciousness lives in your mind, your body, and your spirit, as well as in your relationship with yourself and others. Your health is manifested in how you feel, act, talk, think, and are. Poor health can make each day feel lousy, for health is a reflection of your state of being. Fortunately, it takes only one person to turn things around—and that is you.

The best thing we can do to honor our life is to take care of ourselves, and then our life can be what it is meant to be. When we choose something other than good health for ourselves, we choose a life less than what was planned for us. Poor health compromises our enjoyment of life. You can feel it; it does not hide itself. It makes its presence known to every part of you, because health—whether good or bad—will never lie to you. It will always show itself as it is. Health is connected to the conscious truth with each of us.

It is hard to stay healthy for long without clearing the conscience. A conscience that is not clear cannot foster a healthy mind, and that, in turn, creates an unhealthy body and spirit. Health, therefore, is directly related to truth. If you chose to be healthy, your life will change because you will be facing your issues head-on; no longer will you be running away from them.

It is interesting that unhealthy people often are the most loving, the ones who carry the world on their shoulders, who might carry the load for five or ten others. However, we were not meant to carry the world on our shoulders; if we were, those loving people would be in a perfect paradise. We were meant to carry our own share of life's burdens. So for those people who are trying to get healthy and are chronic caretakers and possible people pleasers: Learn to give to yourself what you have so unselfishly given to others. That is your call to health. Making that change is tough—perhaps the toughest thing you can do—but it will save your health, and ultimately it will save you.

Chapter 4

Commitment and Discipline

Health is a commitment you make to yourself. It entails rising above and beyond your feelings and doing what needs to be done for the sake of your health. It requires a mature attitude, a willingness to put your health first regardless of how you feel, much as you would commit to your family or marriage or your job. In addition, much like a marriage, the beauty and richness of the relationship with health comes out of your commitment to it. Since health is reflected in the relationship one has with themselves upon any given day or time, you can see the glow of a person who enjoys the relationship between their body and themselves. Such a person understands it is not a vanity thing but has to do with the respect one has of being here on the planet and the awesomeness of life. Now, it takes time to get to this place since having been here for a while we have been conditioned so far away from our natural state. Soon this will change; it is changing and evolving right now at this time at speeds very quick. This is happening because consciousness needs to get a hold of us quick because technology or our idea of it is not as great to the evolution of the planet. What is unique about this new understanding of health is we will come to the realization there is no one to cover for us if we fail to hold up our end. Often among our family members or coworkers, there are those who will cover for our weaknesses or our lack of commitment, not so when it comes to our health. There are great healers in the world, absolute gems, thank you God for them, but the reminder is this, we have to do our work to sustain ourselves in the world, the more we do that, the lighter the load on others will be.

Some people are very committed to everything in their lives ... except themselves. If you ask them if they are a committed and disciplined person, they will undoubtedly say yes—but if you ask them if they are committed and disciplined within themselves, they may say no. Staying equally committed to those around you and to yourself may be one of the most difficult things you can do. Therefore, it is important to ask yourself why you are so committed to certain things. Could it be it is time to let go of that commitment and start something new? Is it possible that you are avoiding some problems in your life, and that by staying busy, you are relieved of having to deal with them?

I believe staying in things that are long over do is what causes us to age. Being afraid to let go so new life can be brought in is a natural flow of the life cycle. Being stuck in something for a long time in life is like wearing the same thing all life long. How is that energizing and exciting?.

If we are to stay committed to our health, we must be willing to go through a period of self-discovery and self-realization. Lasting change does not happen without this. The only thing you have to lose is everything that has been weighing you down, so it is worth the effort it takes. It is all about getting rid of what you no longer need, whether it is that false front you have been using for self-protection or the belief that you can wait until retirement to deal with your life issue. Whatever it is Life and or consciousness keeps it all in the holding bin for when we want to deal with it, the sooner the better I say.

Chapter 5

Self-Development/Self-Love

You can train your bodies to become a creature of habit, so when you want to change, it is important that you begin to change "the habit of the creature."

One thing is true: if you're overweight, your issue is not the weight, but the self beneath the weight, the self that has not been heard among the loud noises and demands of the day. If you keep focusing on weight as the cause and effect of your health problems, you will keep coming up short. The cause and effect is the self that has been ignored, the self that has found distraction and escape in things other than the brave action necessary for change to happen, which is to be true to yourself first. When you are true to yourself, you are automatically true to others. Truth is reflected in your relationship with others, but first it must be made manifest in you. The body does not create the health problem, because it is not capable of making a decision on its own; it simply follows the lead of the person inside making decisions on its behalf.

We tend to blame our bodies for our problems because that's where they're most evident, but what's on the outside is a reflection of a problem that goes deeper than is apparent to the eye of the beholder. If we can reach that place deep inside, the holder of that weight, the holder of the physical sadness, we then can start to make the change. But first we must stop blaming our body for our problems and admit that *we* are the problem for our body. Until we can fix that relationship in terms of how we deal with life—how we treat ourselves in response to what's happening in our world—we will continue to be stuck in the same pattern and repeat the same history. So we must be willing to make changes from within, regardless of where our body decides to go, for eventually it will follow. It may take a while—whenever you change your relationship with anything or anyone, there are going to be adjustments to make—but it can be done. Change can be achieved.

Such self-development cannot rushed; it takes effort, patience, and time. It's one of the few things left in life in which technology cannot intervene. That's because self-development is a process of contemplating, understanding, and finally growing. It is the development of your mind and body. Imagine if parents rushed the development of their child, as if to say, "Hurry up and grow up, hurry up and understand and *get it* already," forcing that development along with preexisting beliefs and ideas. Would that child develop a thorough understanding of himself and the world around him?

Opinions vary about the best route to true health, but it stands to reason that if in order to achieve wholeness of mind, body, and spirit, you must first understand how these three very human components work in unison. We're not born blind to these aspects of ourselves; we have just not been made aware of them. Wholeness of mind, body, and spirit was and is the original way of being, the original plan made manifest in our early childhood. Since we lost this sense of wholeness due to the business of living, we are apt to want to rush our self-development along, as we do with many other things in life. However, if we rush our health along, if we force our own agenda and ways upon it, we won't develop a solid understanding of ourselves and our health. It could take eight, ten, even fifteen years to develop good overall mental, physical, emotional, and spiritual health, because humans operate in a fragmented way. Reigning in your understanding and knowledge of yourself is very difficult. In a way, you start out with nothing and build your health from that. Taking control over your health allows you to get back to the beginning of who you really are, because it does not attach itself to concepts of what it should be. You cannot find it wandering around on the outside. Believe me, if you could, you would have found it by now.

Root: 1. essential core: Heart 2. To dig up, turn over or discover and bring to light.

When people decide to get healthy, they tend to buy into whatever is currently being marketed, whether it's books, machines, diet supplements, or foods. That is where we have been conditioned to start any kind of change. So why does this approach not work? People can read books and buy products to learn how to make money, and that works for them. They can go to classes and learn how to become their own boss or read books and learn how to start an entirely new career, with great success. So why is it that this same approach when used in regard to health and fitness has a very low success rate? What's more bewildering is that despite the failures of these get-healthy-quick plans, we keep doing the same thing over again—probably because that's all there is out there. The book covers and the authors change. The exercise machines have different names and features. But overall, the health solutions being marketed to us are repetition at its finest.

Think about the word *root*, defined on the previous page. Anyone who has lived some years has a root inside them. This root is where we hold onto all our truths, all of our pain, all of our fears, and, possibly, our shame. When we try to get healthy each year, when we try and establish new habits and patterns, we only get so far before we quit. And that's frustrating and bewildering. It's hard to understand why we can do so many things and achieve so much in our lives, but we just can't maintain our health. Unfortunately, our bodies cannot tell a lie. Our bodies reveal that root in each of us: our truths, our stories, our grief and suffering.

The world we live in does not create time for us to decompress, to reflect, and to contemplate life, and that time is critical to our health. Most Americans think we can just pick a diet and an exercise routine and everything will be cool, or that if we are losing weight, everything is fine. Well, that is exactly what we have been conditioned to believe—and in fact those things will work for a while. But pretty soon the conditioning wears off and we need something else to carry us the rest of the way. What is that something, and where do we get it? Well, we get it from inside ourselves—the only place we can find the power to get the rest of the way home.

Health does not start on the outside, where we may look for it initially; it starts on the inside. And in order to live in freedom, which health can and will give you, it is important to discern the root cause of your physical condition. Some causes are easy to figure out. If I fell off the roof and broke my hip, for instance, the root cause of my hip condition would be very easy to figure out. On the other hand, if as an adult I developed a fear of deep water, I might not understand the problem until learning from my mother that when I was a child, I fell into deep water and had to be rescued. Knowing the root cause of my fear would be critical to my overcoming it. Without knowing that cause, I might find myself immobilized by fear and unable to understand or solve my phobia.

The point is that what impedes our success, what prevents us from getting past the blocks that mysteriously show up like an unseen veil, is the root inside us. Perhaps someone's words to us when we were younger created the root, or perhaps it stemmed from having lost someone but never having grieved. Those unresolved issues can create a block that keeps you from going forward. So part of taking care of your health is finding out the root cause of your problems. Only you will know about it, and when you look at it now, from an adult perspective and from a different place than you were when the root took hold in you, you can begin healing and loving yourself. Then you'll see for the first time how different things can be.

So why are we still waiting for someone else's better answer or theory? Because we do not want to be the student who does the homework; we just want to be the student who knows it all. Well, we are a nation with a lot of teachers and a lot of students—but not so many people doing the homework, applying the information learned. We seem to be stuck in our approach to health, and we will continue to be stuck if we decide to just absorb information without doing the homework.

What kind of homework? Looking for all the things that can help fix our life situation, such as better ways to lose weight, raise our children, and become healthier. Finding this information takes a student who wants to learn and is then willing to follow through on the information she finds. We all tend to do well at picking up the information we need to make changes in our lives. We know where to find it, and in fact we insist on getting the best, most up-to-date information available, but then we put it on a shelf with all our other self-help books without applying it to our lives. Finding information is just the first part of learning; the second part is putting it into practice. If we don't, we'll feel as though we've failed ourselves.

We are constantly trying to improve our lives. That's human nature. But we must understand that we can't create change through a teacher. It's just as it was in school: your teacher taught, but it was up to you, the student, to learn. The teacher did not get paid to do your work; she got paid to teach, and she graded you according to the effort you put into your studies.

In life, too, there is a lot of homework that we must do to make our way through. There are a lot of teachers out there who have done their homework and are willing to teach us what they know. But they cannot do our homework for us; we must do our own work, make our own way, have our own experiences, and perhaps become teachers ourselves. So when we want to make changes in our health, we have to realize that getting information from doctors is not the same thing as doing the work of changing. The information is available to you, and it's up to you to use it to take on a new life, to learn and practice what it teaches. The effort of learning the information is where your work begins and ends, because once you learn and put into practice one thing, you can master it and then move on to the next.

While most of us are not in the habit of mastering anything, doing so is well worth the effort; it is truly what we are all here for. Anyone can buy anything if they have a lot of money, but no one can buy mastery over the soul and spirit. The truths that can be found from within cannot be bought or sold. They are heavenly and eternal—and they are what we are here to experience. Finding those truths requires letting go of the things we think are so important, trusting our heart of hearts when it tells us there is something missing from this rat race we call "life"—because there is. We can attain our highest potential by mastering certain aspects of ourselves that have taken over our thinking, taken over our lives. If you can learn to master that which once mastered you, then you can begin to experience a new life, unchained and free.

We all have the innate power to change our lives, to change ourselves. Whether you are a man, woman, or child, you are capable of change. Even if you were raised in a family where you did not see a lot of change, where everything stayed the same to the detriment of your life, even if you did not receive proper guidance from those around you, you still have the capability to change yourself.   Yes it takes work, yes it is a process, but what's more important than creating a life you enjoy? If you are living a life of misery, isn't the most important thing you can do right now to work on making things better? Perhaps you feel that you do not have the support to make change. Well, the beautiful thing is that you have more support than you can ever know inside you—and you start the change process by believing that you already have what it takes to achieve your goals. In fact, a lot of people have so much help at their disposal that they actually become dependent on it. They demand ever more help rather than digging deep within themselves to create the change that they're seeking. So remember that the road to change is yours to tread (or walk or run). Whatever it is you decide to do, the road is yours.

If you take on this task of change—whatever that change may be—understand that it will be like doing homework every day. It will become your full-time job, but it will be worth it. It will also require a mindfulness that you've never practiced before, a thought process that you've never tried, and a deep, continuous commitment on your part. Caring is the key to permanent change— wanting and needing something better than you have ever had in your life. No one else should care more about you than you do. That may sound selfish, but it is not. Think about it. If I don't care much about myself, then odds are that I don't love myself much, either. But there are probably plenty of people who love me more than I do, who want more for me than I do ... and what does that say about me? I end up burdening them in a way that is not helpful to either of us. If I love myself less than I should, I probably haven't created the best life for myself, and the less I love myself, the more someone else has to make up the difference. After all, the natural world is about balance, and if I don't take responsibility for taking care of and loving myself, that responsibility will fall to someone else. Wouldn't it be nice to love and care for ourselves as we should, allowing those around us the benefit of a life well lived as well, without our burdens placed upon them? It is selfish *not* to love and take care of yourself.

You can start by cultivating strength and discipline in yourself and your life. Think about the space and time you waste taking care of things that really have no value or meaning—like the overheated arguments about things that have already passed. We spend so much time arguing—and very little time making progress! And we spend a lot of time picking through the details of other people's lives. They are trying to get through life just as we are, but we do not allow them the mistakes they need to make in order to learn and change. If we could all understand that life is a journey, that we are all responsible for doing what we can to develop ourselves, our minds, and our hearts, this world would be in better shape. So as you seek change in your life, don't chase the world. Focus on making yourself better, learn compassion and understanding, and you will find the world a better place in which to live. Then the world will chase you.

Each of us moves in life from the place of a wounded self to that of a healed self. And we can't be healed without first realizing that we are the walking wounded. It is from the perspective of that wounded self that we move and define ourselves, and from which all our decisions are made. Wars are fought as a result of generations of wounds accumulated; they are the actions of people whose souls have not been healed in their own lifetime, whose efforts represent the vain attempt to run away from their wounded selves rather than healing them. Health is not created from the physical body; it doesn't come from nutritious food. It comes from the self that has been healed first. If you try to make your body healthy without healing your wounded self, your physical body cannot be fully healthy and well. On the other hand, a healed self will automatically be drawn toward that which is good for the body.

Attempting to create health without first healing our inner selves is almost impossible, therefore, because it is the wounded self that creates most of the sickness in the body. Think about it: your body was fine, *you* were fine, until someone hurt you, until you suffered loss, until someone was mean to you. When such a thing happens, we keep that hurt deep inside. And then we try and overcome it by overachieving, denying the hurt, or being aggressive toward others. If we could only understand that we were never defined by that hurt—that we were never the insults, we were never the loss or the pain—then we can begin to heal. Instead, we take these hurts personally. We internalize them, and then we end up creating a life out of the wound.

Finding your way back to the self that is true, the self that is you, can be difficult, or it can be easy—no one knows your hurt but you. Stop for a moment and think about the place where you are operating from. Is it your wounded self that is still afraid to stand and recover? You don't have to be in pain; you don't have to be afraid. But you may be in pain—a lot of the time—although you may not know it because you are operating on "automatic pilot." So in order to heal, it's important to discern where you are coming from. You cannot tap into your own potential while covered over in old wounds.

Self-Love

Do you like yourself?

I think this is one of the most important questions to ask and answer at any age.

It's the question you must ask yourself before you go off to "get healthy," because the answer, and how you respond to that answer, can be life-changing—especially if the answer is "No."

Health is for you, and the purpose of health is to turn that "No" into a "Yes." But that can only happen if you are willing to see yourself differently than you ever have before.

You will have to promise to love yourself; that is all Health will ask of you. Poor health stems from a lack of love for the self. Just like anything else, the self soon dies without love. Now *death* is a powerful word, and to some it means not coming back to life ... ever. But the death I am talking about is the death of the spirit, the death of inspiration, of hope, of anything positive. That is what can happen when we do not love ourselves. Love is like a ray of sunshine: it warms the heart and brings smiles. But if we do not love ourselves, we stop enjoying life as we should. The ray of sunshine is gone, and we are left liking ourselves only according to what we do for others, how others feel about or treat us, or whether we did a good job at work. Shouldn't we love ourselves with real love, and not conditional love, which is always fleeting?

Health can return to the body, spirit, mind, and emotions when we start to love ourselves. We were not asked to be born, but here we all are—and there must be a reason. It must mean that life is good, that things are good on earth. When we acknowledge the good inside ourselves, we begin to recognize the good outside us, too.

The soul is empty without love. It ends up starving, and the signs of that starvation are many: depression, laziness, anger, frustration, moodiness, agitation, sadness, and a feeling of being overwhelmed with life. If we don't understand the reason for these feelings, we attribute them to something else, trying this way or that to change them, but it does no good. Just like the stomach knows real food when it is hungry, your soul knows real love when it feels it, and it rejects all the substitutes you may try giving it. The true reason for these negative feelings is that your soul has not been loved and accepted by *you* yet. Consider how much a child needs his parents' love. Food and toys will never work as a substitute for that love. Without it, the child may be getting material things but starving inside for lack of love—waiting and waiting, because that child cannot force his parents to give him what they do not have. But if the parents start to genuinely love the child, for no other reason than a miracle of the heart, the child will come back to life like nothing you have ever seen. Why? Because he finally has received the love he has been waiting for.

It is as if your soul is just waiting for your love. It does not want you to do anything else first—it does not want you to become a success first, it does not want you to become beautiful. It does not care about that, because the soul is love, but it cannot give you that love until you are first willing to love yourself. Here you are, wandering around, doing all sorts of things, but nothing seems to satisfy the emptiness inside you. That's because the emptiness is in your soul, and your soul does not want things. It wants only your love, and in return it will give you life.

We suffer because our soul is suffering; we suffer because we have not yet learned the basic life-giving qualities necessary for happiness. So let us start our change there. Remember, your soul is not looking for anything. It does not need new clothes or a new routine. It just needs you to love it, and once that happens you will have the glorious life you were meant to have. You cannot have a glorious life with a soul that is desperate for your love. You cannot have a meaningful life with a soul that has not yet been claimed. Your soul needs you, and you need it. Every human, every soul needs love.

It is not necessary to *do* much for this to happen, because much good stuff happens automatically once you start to love yourself. Without that love, your attempts to *do* only further burden a soul that doesn't have much to give, because little has been given to it. So before you jump on any bandwagons, love yourself—and then see what happens next.

Doctors are here to talk about our bodies, not the people inside our bodies, yet we keep listening, hoping they can set us free from the problems that we often have created ourselves. Stop looking outside yourself for help, and recognize that it is up to you whether you are free from your problems. As long as you disregard the elephant in the room, good health will continue to elude you. For now, *stop* looking in books to find the answer to your problems; it is already within you. Health is meant to set you free, not to add more burdens to your life, to your mind.

We look to other people for information about our bodies, as if they also can unshackle us and set us free from our problems, but that just is not the case. You hold the secrets to your health; you have the keys to help you. But you will never be able to use them as long as you keep looking outside yourself. The solutions you so desperately want cannot be found in knowing how many pounds you can lose in a week on a certain diet. Nor can they be found in your cholesterol levels. The freedom that you are instinctively—and perhaps subconsciously—seeking cannot be found in anything you have done so far. The freedom you are looking for can be found only in *you*! Your freedom is in you!!

We don't need more books or more doctors to help us. Right now we need to *"know thyself,"* which is the only health remedy we have right now. Nothing else will do, not at this point. What are our children learning from this? Children are smart; they see and know more than we think they do. But we will continue to make a mockery of their lives if we are not willing to deal with the reality of our own. And so it goes.

So far we have taught our children that the answer to any problem is always found outside and not from within. We've set them up for their future—looking outside, of course, for that is how they have been taught to look. We must have the courage to be honest with ourselves so that our children can see better examples around them. That will give them strength to overcome adversity or to practice honesty in action. Instead, such attributes are falling to the wayside, as we are busy doing unnecessary things to avoid facing how we feel about ourselves. The legacy we leave our children can't be changed once we've gone, so be wise in your teaching. And remember that to bring out the best in anyone, you must first see the best in yourself.

Our children have to learn about life, about being human—and they cannot learn any of that when we avoid our own problems. We must start practicing honesty, for ourselves and for them.

The pendulum must find balance now! We have created imbalance from our belief that knowledge alone will keep our problems from happening, solve the ones that we have, or somehow erase the ones that we are afraid to confront. But by avoiding those problems, we are making ourselves sick. Let us get off this crazy train and get on one that is saner. All this knowledge has led to too much focus on our bodies and very little understanding of ourselves.

Chapter 6

The Watcher Is You!

Okay, so we all arrive here by way of a physical body, and within each body is a person. Each body needs a watcher, an advocate, someone inside to look after it, to look out for it. If we do not acknowledge the watcher, the presence in the body that serves as its protection, who else will be assigned to that task? Who takes that place? Well, if no one claims the role of watching over your body, someone or something else will for sure. For if you aren't home, something will want to get in and take over the position of homeowner, whether it's a drug, toxic foods, or massive overstimulation of the brain, mind, or body—anybody or anything in reach of your eyes or ears has the chance to take over if you are not home. That is what has taken place: there has been a void of ownership within your body, so it has become fully receptive to anyone wanting to sell whatever you "feel" you want.

We have created substitute owners within our bodies. They seek only what feels good—and that's dangerous, for then there is no one inside the body looking out for its best interest. We are all having fun while not being present within our own bodies. Our bodies are without owners that watch over them and make sure that what they are putting into them is good, advocates who are home 24/7 because they know that without them, their bodies do not have a chance in this world. The body needs a vigilant owner. Without one, it is powerless over the societal deluge of addictive medicines, food, alcohol, and overstimulation.

Things do and will "just happen" if we are never home to keep watch. Why do you think that children are not left alone? Because without an adult watching over them, they will get into everything; they are not capable of looking out for themselves. In the same way, our bodies need the presence of an adult. If we see our bodies as young children who need someone to watch over them, we can begin to understand that throughout life we will never outgrow the role of owners and watchers of our own bodies.

We tend to assume that because we are able to make a living or raise a family, we have it all together. Well, if we're neglecting our body, then we don't. Our body needs us to be home, to watch out for its best interests, in order for it to live a good and long life. When we forget that responsibility, we fall into health trouble. Be home for your body. Without you at home and in control, too much can happen that is not good, not worth the sleep, not worth the escape. Health happens only when the owner is home. If the owner wants good health but is never home, who is going to be there? Who is going to watch and pay attention? Who is going to be responsible for the body? Instead of paying attention to everything that is happening outside, stay home. That alone can be the answer to your health problems. Be your body's advocate, its loving owner. For without you, there is not much chance for change.

Chapter 7

What Provokes and Creates Change?

Often when people decide to get healthier, they approach the task in a half-hearted way—and the end result is just that: half-hearted, half-finished, half-planned. Eventually, the goal just fades away.

Health needs to be approached in a way that provokes the change you want to see. How do you do this? Well, when you provoke something long enough, it eventually gives in to you.

Let me clarify. If you begin with a half-hearted approach to your health, you have put yourself in charge of something already doomed to failure. No wonder you don't make it! Your approach needs to change in order for things to turn out differently. Good health is what you want, right? In order to get what you want, then, you must first make friends with it. Remember, Health is smart. Up until now, you may have viewed health as your nemesis, your pain in the butt. Well, if you continue to think in those terms, it will constantly elude you, for we tend to push our enemies away. If you look at Health as something frightening or unachievable, then quite possibly it will not happen for you. On the other hand, if you look at Health as something friendly, something you want to get to know, something you are capable of getting, then maybe you'll get somewhere with it.

When you're on a mission to change, it's important to understand that the mind plays an important part in the process. There are several questions you must consider. How do you want to change? How do you begin that change? Why do some people change while others don't? What is the common denominator of change?

The common denominator of change is the ability to master the mind. The decline of physical discipline and strength, the softening of passion for life, is due to the lack of mastery of the mind. If you allow a two-year-old access to whatever she wants, whenever she wants it, disciplining her only occasionally, she will not stay disciplined very long. After all, she has been the master over the adult most of the time. And in fact, it is much easier to spoil a child than to discipline her, but that will not result in a healthy, well-adjusted child. In the same way, creating healthy change inside yourself requires regular discipline, mental exercise practiced throughout the day. I call it *mind-sitting*.

Yes, mind-sitting is what you do to create change, and what you keep doing until that change has been established within your body. And yes, it is constant work; after all, you're reversing damage from years of neglect. The mind under your watch has become very spoiled. It has operated without regulations, free to do whatever it wants, when it wants. It will continue in its quest for satisfaction, so that you must constantly attend to it. The experience is kind of like babysitting that two-year-old, but it is *mind-sitting* a two-year-old, instead. It's not fun. It's hard work. But it must be done in order for your mind to mature so that someday you can trust it.

One thing to watch out for is knowing when the mind is "grown up." You do not want to micromanage your mind; that just creates tension, a false need to control your thoughts. It is not necessary to overreact to your thoughts. So stay alert to the signs that your mind has matured. There will be changes in your physical appearance, improvements in your attitude toward yourself and others, and a sweet, kind dialogue inside your own mind.

The maturation of the mind—its evolution from child to teenager to adult— is quite an interesting thing, so just maintaining objectivity while the process is happening is a good idea. Once you've noticed drastic changes in your mind and your physical appearance, you should begin trusting your mind more. Let it go. Establish a new, healthy relationship with your mind by giving it what it needs, which is the freedom to be. The mind that respects you for what you have done to discipline it, and it will respect you even more if you allow it to be what it was meant to be in the first place. Allow it the freedom to help you live. Don't suppress it out of fear that it will become spoiled; that won't happen again once you understand how it works and respect its capabilities. And recognize that it has a job to do for you, just like your heart and your lungs.

Now, it might sound to you as if "mastering the mind" is a matter of control. It is not. Basically, it is a matter of love. It is caring for yourself enough to say, *No, I do not need everything that I want. No, it is not healthy for my mind to be in charge of me or my life. My mind is not that smart—it's great for storage, but it is not so good at leading. It is good at thinking about things, recalling things, but when it is spoiled and undisciplined, it thinks it's the boss, which it is not. It is a good support, though.*

Chapter 8

Taking Physical Action

Fitness creates inner development.

When you are ready to get fit, when you are ready to start to take better care of yourself than ever before, there are some things that you may need to know.

To begin with, you will be called to do *more* then you expect. Up until now, you may have viewed health and fitness as an external process. You plan, buy, and prepare the right food. You tour the gym, sign up for a membership, and go work out.

The truth of the matter is that health and fitness is all about inner development, and that's tough work. You become out of shape and overweight because you've forgotten that it is your responsibility to take care of yourself. Once that lightbulb comes on over your head, change will begin to happen. You'll begin wanting to take good care of yourself, until it becomes second nature. Yes, it can happen.

Inner development is what happens naturally, through the process of taking care of you.

The Super Bowl is not won on physical strength alone. It is won by each player's willingness to develop and understand himself and the game. No play goes unnoticed as players review film in preparation for the contest: they analyze, they scrutinize, and in order for them to develop to their very best, they must take the good with the bad and look at the whole picture—even when it is hard to look at. But in the end, if they are willing to put their pride aside and study the film objectively, accepting what they see and moving forward in a positive way, they have a better chance of winning. In that room, there is no running away, there is no hiding, and the camera never lies. So in your quest for better health, you be the coach and let your conscience be the camera. If you are willing to be strong, willing to keep moving forward with a fearless and courageous attitude, you will be on your way to winning your own Super Bowl.

Like football, health and fitness are not just played on the field but practiced off the field, as well. It is all aspects of the game—not just what's seen on the outside—that creates a win.

Health Can Be a Battle of Wills

Health can be a battle of wills. While you may want it, your will to change may be locked somewhere inside you, battling to stay alive. We live most of our lives unaware that we are going against the will of the body and toward the will of the self. So to venture off into the land of health is to change your will, so to speak, and that's a challenge. It's hard to overcome obstacles that don't want to move. Imagine, for example, that you're the parent of an adult child who decides to live at home way past the time when he should have moved out. You might want him to move out, which is reasonable—it is your home, after all, and he is an adult. The problem is that you've allowed him to live there as an adult for so long that it is difficult for you to make an argument for why he should leave now. Therein lies the battle of wills: one will says, *If you wanted me to leave, you should have done it a long time ago,* and the other says, *This is my home, I have the right to decide who stays here, and it's your time to leave.* As a parent, you have been speaking out of both sides of your mouth in your actions and in your relationship, possibly to keep the peace. You love your son, and he knows that. So where do you draw the line? It is a tough thing to do, battling the will of someone you love, changing a situation you've put up with for so long. It's hard to go through the difficult stage of making a stand and sticking to it.

So when you want health, your will that you have allowed to stay for so long—your will that's long on fun and feeling good, and short on everything else—is going to argue, kick, and scream. And it must come to an understanding that the will of Health must take precedence in order for positive change to happen. Before, the order of the day was *your* will; now it is the will of Health. It is difficult, but for change to take place, you must relax your will and favor the will of your health. Ultimately, Health will allow you true freedom, because it does not want to argue and battle, but for you to reach health, your will has to bend. You may not know what to expect because you have never done this before, but if you use your mind as a tool, setting yourself up for success by just thinking about health, you will move in that direction; your thoughts will gradually change your will. The going may not be perfect, and that's okay. The simple fact that you have health on your mind will allow your will to change. It takes time, but just be patient and keep your mind on the goal, and your body will follow.

We are destined in life not to know our bodies, but to know ourselves. And in our quest for health, we will in due time and with perseverance come to know ourselves.

Health is dealing with life on a reality basis. So it will not allow you to whitewash over anything that you may not want to deal with, because if you want to play that game you will get less of what health has to give. Just be honest with yourself, as you body is very forgiving however; it makes for a horrible place to confiscate what you do not want to admit yourself. You are the person in the body that has to stand up to the past in order to be healthy for your future.

Each person is the answer to their own health condition. For that condition would not exist without the choices of the one made behind the condition. We cannot keep working any longer for the answer, it cannot be found outside of the person. The condition of someone's health within their physical bodies happened by the choices that they make and have made previously. Unless the person decides on changing the choices that they make the condition of the body cannot change. Unless the person decides to make healthier decisions, the health condition will continue to decline.

We cannot continue to keep addressing the food, we must address ourselves, and how it is that we are taking care of ourselves. We must address the question within ourselves as to why, which each person has the answer to, and then go from there. We must admit that we need to learn how to take care of ourselves, and them the care begins. Before that, you have a person that continues to inject food without practicing any form of exercise, all because they do not know how important it is yet to take care of their health. Our bodies are what hold the continuation of the quality of our lives. If the quality of our lives seem less the adequate, it is only because out health within out body has been compromised. We must come to understand, that in order to have a life that is energized and clear, we must take care of the organs that can create that condition. Good health is found in our choice to take care of ourselves, each day. Not just because an event is coming up and we want to look good. IF a person can learn and get the truth to take care of them, and keep it simple that way, they will have found the key to a happy life. Life takes care of the person who takes care of themselves. And I do not mean monetarily, or by having more things, what I mean by that statement, is that when you take care of your body, your mind becomes clear, you have a confidence in life that you did not have before, you tend to gain an appreciation for life, because you can now sense something more to life that was not there before.

What could be more important then to take care of your health, when in doing so, the quality of the rest of your life is effective instantly each moment.

We cannot disassociate ourselves with our health anymore, we must face the music. We wake up tired and sluggish and then we do not bother to understand and learn where that is coming from, we have spent so much time ignoring ourselves, that now we do not even realize it. With the prescription drugs on the rise, and all of these people going in for surgery, they are not learning anything about themselves, they are not even thinking about learning why it is that they are in the poor health that they are in. the answer is not given by a Doctor, it is within ourselves. It is important to take the time to investigate why it is that you are in the condition that you are in. Yes we have doctors, and we need doctors, but the truth of the matter is, is that we are the sole owners of our bodies. We are the ones that should be held accountable for the way that we take care of ourselves, and if we lean too heavily on the doctors we do not find the real answer within ourselves. For instance if you suffer from depression, and the doctor knows this, he is not there to have a long conversation about why you have depression, so just because you have some medication, does not mean that you have found the cause of the depression. you must investigate the cause before you go to the doctor, see first what it is that is the reason for this conditon.You will be doing yourself a big favor. We all must deal with issues from time to time; it is not the end of the world. It is o.k. But let's deal with our health in the most effective way. Through eating foods that are not conventionally made, is a start, by exercise is another key factor, and as you do these things, then other things become clear to you and that is the beauty of taking care of yourself. Where everything that you may have been doing, was pushing down and trying to hide how you felt about something, is now revealed. Because things are clear. We cannot reach clarity with a mind that is foggy and a body that is clogged, where energy is at a low level. So working through from mud and slug with our bodies, towards clear water takes time. But it is the most important thing that you can do for yourself.

We need our body's period, so it is important to take care of you all day long. Now, that does not mean anything but be aware of what you are putting into your body, and exercise, that is it, there is no need to be consumed with anything. Just take care of your body, so that it can take care of you in a very beautiful way. With high energy, beauty, brightness. It is about being alive. If we pack our bodies with food that is "dead" We feel practically "dead" If we pack our bodies with "life" then we feel alive, that is the key. Just try it out, it is not a diet, it is not anything but simplicity.

www.ingramcontent.com/pod-product-compliance
Lightning Source LLC
Chambersburg PA
CBHW020351290526
45785CB00005B/2230